Special Tests of the Cardiopulmonary, Vascular and Gastrointestinal Systems

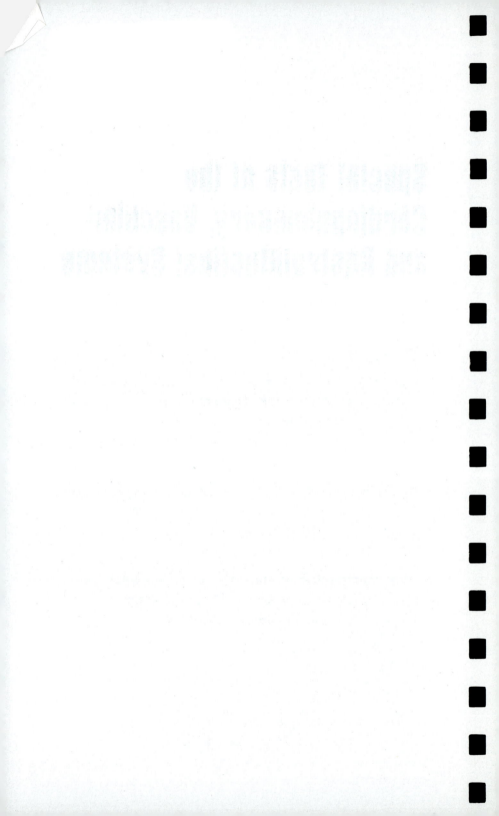

Special Tests of the Cardiopulmonary, Vascular and Gastrointestinal Systems

Dennis G. O'Connell, PT, PhD, CSCS, FACSM
Professor and Endowed Chair
Department of Physical Therapy
Hardin-Simmons University
Abilene, Texas

Janelle K. O'Connell, PT, PhD, DPT, ATC, LAT
Professor, Department of Physical Therapy
Hardin-Simmons University
Abilene, Texas

Martha R. Hinman, PT, EdD, CEEAA
Professor, Department of Physical Therapy
Hardin-Simmons University
Abilene, Texas

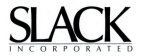

www.slackbooks.com

ISBN: 978-1-55642-966-8

Copyright © 2011 by SLACK Incorporated

Photography by Dr. Tim Chandler, EdD - Higher Education. Director Media Production, Associate Professor Communication, Hardin-Simmons University, Abilene, TX.

Published by: SLACK Incorporated
                       6900 Grove Road
                       Thorofare, NJ 08086 USA
                       Telephone: 856-848-1000
                       Fax: 856-848-6091
                       www.slackbooks.com

Contact SLACK Incorporated for more information about other books in this field or about the availability of our books from distributors outside the United States.

Library of Congress Cataloging-in-Publication Data

O'Connell, Dennis G.
 Special tests of the cardiopulmonary, vascular, and gastrointestinal systems / Dennis G. O'Connell, Janelle K. O'Connell, Martha R. Hinman.
    p. ; cm.
 Includes bibliographical references and index.
 ISBN 978-1-55642-966-8
 1. Function tests (Medicine) 2. Cardiopulmonary system--Diseases--Diagnosis. 3. Cardiovascular system--Diseases--Diagnosis. 4. Gastrointestinal system--Diseases--Diagnosis. I. O'Connell, Janelle K. II. Hinman, Martha R. III. Title.
 [DNLM: 1. Physical Examination--methods. 2. Diagnostic Techniques, Cardiovascular. 3. Diagnostic Techniques, Digestive System. 4. Diagnostic Techniques, Respiratory System. 5. Exercise Test--methods. WB 205 O18s 2011]
 RC71.8.O34 2011
 616.1'075--dc22

                                    2010024032

Last digit is print number: 10 9 8 7 6 5 4 3 2 1

DEDICATION

To our Father God, and all those who utilize His gifts and graces as shepherds, servants, and stewards.

CONTENTS

x   Contents

ACKNOWLEDGMENTS

Over the course of my educational and professional career, several individuals have inspired and encouraged me to take on new challenges. They include Charles Busuttil, Drs. Edward Howley, Fred Andres, and William Gould. Their passion and drive in the pursuit of excellence has encouraged and inspired me. They are true educators, true gentlemen, and most outstanding role models.

My collaborator, colleague, and friend, Dr. Martha Hinman, provided expertise on a number of special tests, reduced several tables, and reviewed the book. My friends and faculty colleagues, Drs. Brewer, Friberg, Garrett, Palmer, and Rutland, as well as my students, excite and challenge me on a daily basis to become a better teacher, writer, collaborator, and clinician.

The Hardin-Simmons University classes of 2007-2009 were extremely helpful and often located a variety of manuscripts that may have been used within this text. My favorite librarian, Mrs. Leta Tillman, has obtained hundreds of manuscripts that have been used to create this work. Mrs. Karen Freeland and Mrs. Ann Jones have been helpful in countless ways. I greatly appreciate the time and effort of model, Mr. Pete Hinman, as well as models Dr. Nikki Powers, Mr. Tanner Zimmerman and Ms. Loretta Pugh. Dr. Tim Chandler volunteered his time and expertise providing all photographic images. At SLACK Incorporated, Brien Cummings and Debbie Steckel have consistently cajoled, prodded, and provided support.

My parents, George and Grace O'Connell, and in-laws, Carl and Joann Pohlman, along with our extended families, have always been a source of encouragement. Of course, my greatest encourager is my loving wife and colleague, Dr. Janelle O'Connell. In addition to authoring the Abdominal Evaluation section and organizing all figures and photographs, she repeatedly reviewed the entire text and attended to numerous details. While I suffer from "AADD"—or "author attention deficit disorder"—her exceptional organizational ability and pragmatism made this text a reality. I hope our efforts encourage our children, Evan, Cameron, and Keelan, as well as our students, to appreciate the benefits and importance of life-long learning.

Dennis G. O'Connell, PT, PhD, CSCS, FACSM

ABOUT THE AUTHORS

Dennis G. O'Connell, PT, PhD, CSCS, FACSM is a founding member of Hardin-Simmons University Department of Physical Therapy. He serves as a professor and the Shelton-Lacewell Endowed Chair. He is an adjunct professor at the Rocky Mountain University of Health Professions in Provo, Utah.

Dr. O'Connell received his Bachelor of Science in Physical Education from Manhattan College, his Master of Arts and PhD in Exercise Physiology from Kent State University and the University of Toledo, respectively. He obtained a second Bachelor of Science degree in Physical Therapy from The University of Texas Health Science Center at San Antonio.

Dr. O'Connell has 30 years of experience as an exercise physiologist and 15 years as a physical therapist. His clinical experience has centered on patients with cardiac, pulmonary, and musculoskeletal disorders, and ergonomic issues. In addition to providing pro bono services on-campus, he and his wife, Janelle, created HSU PT Ministries and have served with their students in Guatemala, Mexico, and Abilene, TX.

Janelle K. O'Connell, PT, PhD, DPT, ATC, LAT is a founding member of Hardin-Simmons University Department of Physical Therapy where she currently serves as professor and department head.

Dr. O'Connell received her Bachelor of Science in Education from Central Michigan University, her Master of Arts in Exercise Physiology from Kent State University, and her PhD in Health Promotion from the University of Toledo. She has earned an entry-level MPT and a DPT from Hardin-Simmons University.

Dr. O'Connell has 14 years of experience as a physical therapist and has been an athletic trainer for 31 years. As an athletic trainer, Dr. O'Connell has worked in high school and collegiate sports and in athletic training education. She is a Certified Exercise Expert for Aging Adults and enjoys working with the elderly.

Martha R. Hinman, PT, EdD, CEEAA is a professor in the Hardin-Simmons University Department of Physical Therapy and an adjunct professor at the University of Alabama at Birmingham and the University of Indianapolis. Dr. Hinman received her Bachelor of Science in Physical Therapy and her Master of Health Education from the Medical College of Georgia and earned her EdD in Allied Health Education and Administration at the University of Houston. Dr.

Hinman's 34 years of experience as a physical therapist have focused in the areas of wound care, orthopedics, and geriatric wellness. She is a Certified Exercise Expert for Aging Adults and has expertise in the assessment of fall and fracture risk in the elderly. Dr. Hinman has been involved in physical therapy education for 30 years and has served as an educational consultant and accreditation reviewer for numerous physical therapy programs across the United States.

PREFACE

During the past 15 years, I have been fortunate to teach courses in cardiovascular and pulmonary patient management and management of patients with systemic diseases to physical therapy students. During that time period, the US health care system has undergone considerable change and sweeping changes are likely ahead. While few legislators and few third-party payers have the foresight to encourage and reward preventive services, it has always been my belief that "the best medicine is prevention." While much of clinical medicine, nursing, and allied health are directed at managing disease, what if practitioners took aim at preventing medical catastrophe via a careful evaluation of each patient with simple but valid, reliable, sensitive, and specific tests and measures? As an example, my father was diagnosed with an abdominal aneurysm on a routine physical examination. A physical therapy colleague identified a suspicious (ultimately cancerous) skin lesion on a cardiologist-friend for which he was successfully diagnosed and treated. While prevention through careful evaluation is the goal of most practitioners, a brief, "how-to" guide to clinically important physiological systems with supportive evidence was lacking.

The work of Dr. Jeff G. Konin, author of *Special Tests for Orthopedic Examination* was quite impressive and, upon discussion, he encouraged me to pursue authoring a text that would complement his fine work. In the interim, Dr. James R. Scifers created *Special Tests for Neurologic Examination*, another outstanding and useful manual. I believe the current text completes what I consider an important group of works that will aid health care professionals in the detection and management of injury and disease.

In summary, it is my hope that readers will use this text as they learn or review evaluation of structures within the chest, abdomen, and lower extremities. For those who believe exercise is an important preventive tool, a brief section on submaximal exercise evaluation and exercise prescription has also been included. Because no work is perfect or complete, I encourage communication as I endeavor to strive for these goals. Please contact me at bookspublishing@wyanokegroup.com to share your ideas on ways to improve and add to future editions of this book.

Dennis G. O'Connell, PT, PhD, CSCS, FACSM
Professor and Endowed Chair
Department of Physical Therapy
Hardin-Simmons University

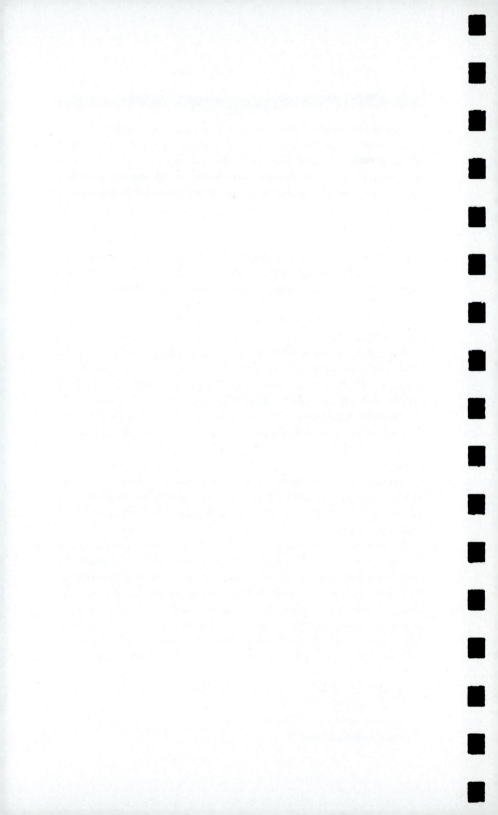

FOREWORD

Special Tests of the Cardiopulmonary, Vascular and Gastrointestinal Systems is a text that is long overdue. The authors have succeeded in amalgamating a variety of resources into one user-friendly, concise volume. Noteworthy is the use of a consistent format in the description of each test with well-conceived figures clarifying patient position and clinician hand placement. Additionally helpful is the clear presentation of normal and positive findings following each test description. Strategically designated tables also aid the reader by providing normative data and expanded explanations. The final chapter and appendices are especially useful to those who often search a plethora of sources to locate a desired cardiopulmonary exercise-testing protocol. Combine all of this with the step-by-step descriptions of equipment calibration and *Special Tests of the Cardiopulmonary, Vascular and Gastrointestinal Systems* becomes a requisite personal library addition for clinicians and educators alike. Kudos to the authors and the publisher for filling this gap in the special test literature.

Donald K. Shaw, PT, PhD, FAACVPR
Associate Professor
Physical Therapy Program
Midwestern University
Glendale, Arizona

INTRODUCTION

To state that clinicians and students are busy is a gross understatement. Clinicians must be able to survive in a world where reimbursement continues to be reduced and per-visit clinician-patient contact decreases. Subsequently, it is imperative to make proper decisions, diagnoses, and referrals in a cost-effective manner. This brief text has been developed for the health care provider who is seeking to use the best, currently available tests and measures. Additionally, harried students, faced with the impossible task of reading hundreds of pages nightly, will benefit from this handy manual, which concisely outlines how to perform a variety of cardiovascular, pulmonary, abdominal, and exercise tests.

Our purpose has been to create a user-friendly text. As such, it has been organized into cardiovascular, pulmonary, gastrointestinal, peripheral vascular, and submaximal exercise evaluation sections. Specific tests and measures are outlined in each section. Additionally, helpful appendices as well as an index are included. The reader will note the generous use of photographs to illustrate the actions describing how each test is administered. Text has been kept to a minimum so that clinicians can turn to a specific page, review the text and actions, and adequately perform the assessment. Because evidence-based practice is best practice, supportive evidence is listed as often as possible, usually in the special considerations section.

Every effort has been made to include references addressing the validity, reliability, sensitivity, and specificity of each test when available. Great difficulty was encountered in this endeavor; however, the process continues.

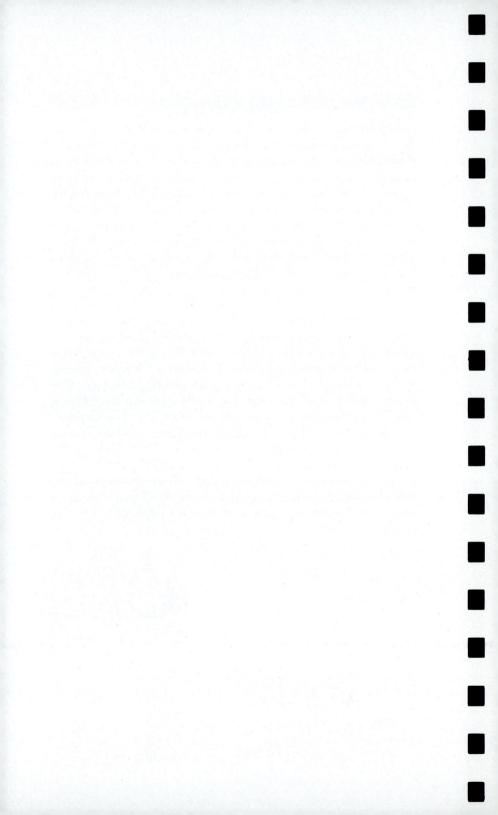

Section

ONE

Examination of the Cardiovascular System

CARDIOVASCULAR DISEASE RISK FACTORS

ACTION

- Obtain oral/written family and risk factor history, or peruse client record for risk factor information.

Table 1-1

CORONARY ARTERY DISEASE RISK FACTORS[1,2]

Family history	• Myocardial infarction, stent, coronary artery bypass graft, OR
	• Sudden death in father or other first-degree male relative <55 years of age, OR
	• Sudden death in mother or other first-degree female relative <65 years of age
Hypertension	• Systolic ≥140 mm Hg or diastolic ≥90 mm Hg, OR
	• Confirmed on 2 separate occasions, OR
	• Taking antihypertensive medication
Dyslipidemia	• HDL ≤40 mg/dL or on lipid-lowering medication, OR
	• LDL cholesterol ≥130 mg/dL, OR
	• Total cholesterol ≥200 mg/dL (if LDL results are unavailable)
Cigarette smoking	• Current smoker or recent quitter (≤6 months)
Impaired fasting glucose	• Fasting blood glucose ≥100 mg/dL on 2 separate occasions
Obesity	• Body mass index ≥30 kg/m^2, OR
	• Waist circumference/hip circumference ≥88% for women, ≥95% for men, OR
	• Waist circumference ≥88 cm for women, ≥102 cm for men
Sedentary lifestyle	• Adults not participating 5 days/week in 30 minutes of moderate aerobic physical activity

Adapted from American College of Sports Medicine. *ACSM's Guidelines for Exercise Testing and Prescription.* 7th ed. Philadelphia, PA: Lippincott Williams & Wilkins; 2005, and Wilson PW, D'Agostino RB, Levy D, Belanger AM, Silbershatz H, Kannel WB. Prediction of coronary heart disease using risk factor categories. *Circulation.* 1998;97:1837-1847.

O'Connell DG, O'Connell JK, Hinman MR.
Special Tests of the Cardiopulmonary, Vascular and Gastrointestinal Systems (pp 2-38).
© 2011 SLACK Incorporated

SPECIAL CONSIDERATIONS

- Prevalence of cardiovascular disease is greater in men vs women and greater in both groups with increasing age[2]
- LDL-C, total cholesterol, HDL-C, blood pressure, and gender are used in the Framingham equations[2] and predict risk of developing angina pectoris, myocardial infarction, or coronary disease over the course of 10 years[3]
- Framingham data primarily describe risk factors in white men and women and may not be generalizable to other ethnic groups
- Every effort should be made to reduce risk factors through behavioral changes (exercise and nutrition) and medication as needed

REFERENCES

1. American College of Sports Medicine. *ACSM's Guidelines for Exercise Testing and Prescription*. 7th ed. Philadelphia, PA: Lippincott, Williams & Wilkins; 2005.
2. Wilson PW, D'Agostino RB, Levy D, Belanger AM, Silbershatz H, Kannel WB. Prediction of coronary heart disease using risk factor categories. *Circulation*. 1998;97:1837-1847.
3. Estimate of 10-Year Risk for Coronary Heart Disease: Framingham Point Scores. http://www.nhlbi.nih.gov/guidelines/cholesterol/risk_tbl.htm. Accessed March 18, 2010.

CARDIOVASCULAR
SYSTEM

HEART RATE–RESTING (ADULTS)

TEST POSITION

- Seated or supine; arm relaxed and supported by a comfortable surface or the examiner (Figure 1-1)

ACTION

- Index and middle fingertip pads lightly palpate the desired pulse points
- Radial or carotid pulse most commonly assessed; other pulse points include: temporal, brachial, femoral, popliteal, tibialis anterior, dorsalis pedis
- Count number of beats in 60 seconds
    - ✧ Shorter duration measurements increase error

        60-second count ± 1 beat/minute
        30-second count ± 2 beats/minute
        15-second count ± 4 beats/minute
        10-second count ± 6 beats/minute

NORMAL FINDINGS

- 60-100 beats/min[1]
- <60 beats/minute in aerobically trained

POSITIVE FINDINGS

- Tachycardia (>100 beats/minute)
    - ✧ Suggestive of anemia, hyperthyroidism, fever, anxiety[2]
- Bradycardia (<60 beats/minute)
    - ✧ Possibly due to sinus bradycardia, second-degree or complete heart block[2]
- Skipped or extra beats
    - ✧ Premature atrial, nodal, or ventricular beats, sinus arrhythmia, second-degree heart block—Mobitz Type I[2]

SPECIAL CONSIDERATIONS

- Resting heart rate is often low in aerobically trained individuals
- Resting heart rate is often elevated during illness or following repetitive days of heavy work
- In hypertensive adults, single heart rate measurements made in the clinic were significantly higher (3.8 ± 8.0 beats/min) than

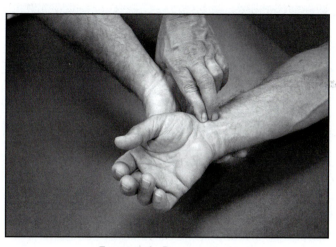

FIGURE 1-1. RADIAL PULSE.

24-hour heart rate averages and daytime average heart rates
(1.1 ± 9.1 beats/min)[3]

- Clinic and ambulatory heart rates were lower in men vs women
  and higher in subjects without cardiovascular complications[3]
- An apical pulse rate may be obtained by placing a stethoscope
  head at the level of the fourth and fifth intercostal space at the
  midclavicular line

REFERENCES

1. Bickley LS. *Bates' Pocket Guide to Physical Examination and History Taking*. 9th ed.
   Baltimore, MD: Lippincott Williams & Wilkins; 2007.
2. Willms JL, Schneiderman H, Algranati PS. *Physical Diagnosis: Bedside Evaluation
   of Diagnosis and Function*. Baltimore, MD: Williams & Wilkins; 1994.
3. Palatini P, Thijs L, Staessen JA, et al. Predictive value of clinic and ambulatory heart rate for mortality in elderly subjects with systolic hypertension.
   Arch Intern Med. 2002;162:2313-2321.

HEART RATE—RESTING (INFANTS-ADOLESCENTS)

TEST POSITION
- Resting: supine or seated

ACTION
- Lightly palpate radial, brachial, or carotid pulse
- Other pulse points include temporal, femoral, popliteal, tibialis anterior, dorsalis pedis
- Count number of beats in 60 seconds (see guidelines for adults)

NORMAL FINDINGS[1]
- Resting heart rate declines with age
- Large standard deviations that lessen with age

Table 1-2
NORMAL FINDINGS

Age	Average Heart Rate
Birth-1 yr	140-115
1-4 yrs	110-105
6-18 yrs	95-82

Adapted from Holloway BW. *Stat Facts: The Clinical Pocket Reference for Nurses.* Philadelphia, PA: F.A. Davis; 1996, and Bickley LS, Szilagyi PG. *Bates' Guide to Physical Examination and History Taking.* 9th ed. Philadelphia, PA: Lippincott Williams & Wilkins; 2007.

POSITIVE FINDINGS[2]
See Table 1-3 on following page.

SPECIAL CONSIDERATIONS
- Resting heart rate varies from day to day
- Sinus arrhythmia, resulting in an increased heart rate with inspiration and decreased HR with expiration, is a normal variant
- Resting heart rate may elevate during illness or following repetitive days of heavy work

Table 1-3

ABNORMAL FINDINGS

Group	Diagnosis	Possible Pathology
Infant	Tachycardia (180 beats/min)	Anxiety or sudden rapid rate requiring treatment[2]
Infant	Bradycardia	Serious underlying disease[2]
Children	Tachycardia	Anemia, atrial fibrillation, congenital heart disease, fever, pain, sinus tachycardia, dehydration
Children	Bradycardia	Numerous, including anaphylaxis, allergic reaction, sick sinus syndrome, or heart block
Adolescent	Tachycardia	Abnormal beats (premature atrial or ventricular contractions), pacemaker pathologies (sick sinus syndrome, complete heart block), aberrant pacemakers (supraventricular or ventricular tachycardia), or abnormal conduction pathways (Wolff-Parkinson-White syndrome)
Adolescent	Bradycardia	Sinoatrial node or conduction pathway problems, hypothermia, heart damage

Adapted from Holloway BW. *Stat Facts: The Clinical Pocket Reference for Nurses.* Philadelphia, PA: F.A. Davis; 1996, and Bickley LS, Szilagyi PG. *Bates' Guide to Physical Examination and History Taking.* 9th ed. Philadelphia, PA: Lippincott Williams & Wilkins; 2007.

REFERENCES

1. Holloway BW. *Stat Facts: The Clinical Pocket Reference for Nurses.* Philadelphia, PA: F.A. Davis; 1996.
2. Bickley LS, Szilagyi PG. *Bates' Guide to Physical Examination and History Taking.* 9th ed. Philadelphia, PA: Lippincott Williams & Wilkins; 2007.

PULSES

TEST POSITION
- Resting, supine, or seated position (examiner choice)

ACTION
- Index and middle fingertips palpate unilateral pulse for 60 seconds
- Note rate, rhythm, and force (amplitude)
- Compare right and left sides

Table 1-4

PULSE AMPLITUDE AND CAUSATION

	Force (Amplitude)	*Possible Causative Factors*
3+	Increased, full, bounding	Exercise, anxiety, fever, anemia, hyperthyroidism
2+	Normal	
1+	Weak	Shock, peripheral arterial disease
0	Absent	Obstruction, death

Adapted from Jarvis C. *Physical Examination and Health Assessment.* 5th ed. St. Louis, MO: Saunders-Elsevier; 2008.

NORMAL FINDINGS
- Rate (60 to 100 beats/min), regular rhythm, normal amplitude

POSITIVE FINDINGS[1]
- Abnormal rate and/or rhythm (see Table 1-5 on following page.)

SPECIAL COMMENTS/CONSIDERATIONS
- Pulses should be assessed in a warm room
- Carotid pulses assessed unilaterally only, with simultaneous cardiac auscultation
- Do not rub or press hard enough to cause occlusion
- Both radial and ulnar pulses may not be found in each upper extremity
- Brachial pulses preferred for measurements in infants

Table 1-5

PULSES AND THEIR LOCATIONS

Pulse	Location
Temporal	Over temporal bone, lateral to eyebrow
Carotid	Medial to sternocleidomastoid, just below angle of mandible
Radial	Proximal to carpals, lateral side of ventral forearm
Ulnar	Proximal to carpals, medial side of ventral forearm
Brachial	Medial humerus between biceps and triceps, or inferior to biceps insertion in antecubital fossa
Femoral	Below inguinal ligament and approximately half-way between the anterior superior iliac spine and symphysis pubis
Popliteal	Within popliteal fossa behind knee. May be palpated with client supine or prone with knee flexed
Tibialis anterior	Posterior and slightly inferior to medial malleolus
Dorsalis pedis	Over the dorsum of the foot, often between first and second extensor tendons

- Popliteal pulse is slightly lateral to midline, difficult to palpate, and may be ignored if distal pulses are palpable
- Tibialis posterior and dorsalis pedis pulses are difficult to palpate
  - ✧ Inability to palpate either or both on ipsilateral foot does not always indicate pathology
  - ✧ Absent posterior tibial pulses are best single predictor of lower extremity occlusive arterial disease
  - ✧ Pedal pulses are absent in ~12% of healthy clients
- Use a Doppler if pulses cannot be palpated

REFERENCE

1. Jarvis C. *Physical Examination and Health Assessment.* 5th ed. St. Louis, MO: Saunders-Elsevier; 2008.

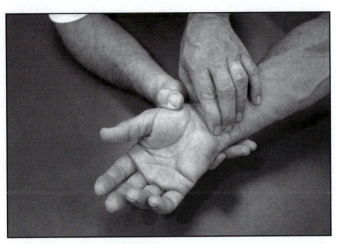

FIGURE 1-2. ULNAR PULSE.

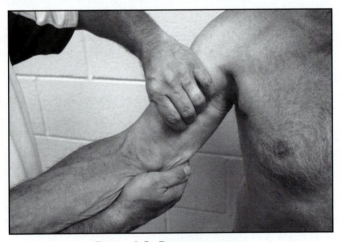

FIGURE 1-3. BRACHIAL PULSE.

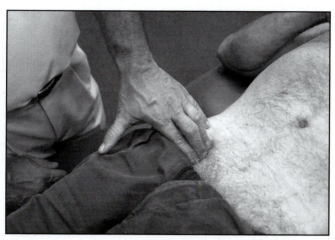

FIGURE 1-4. FEMORAL PULSE.

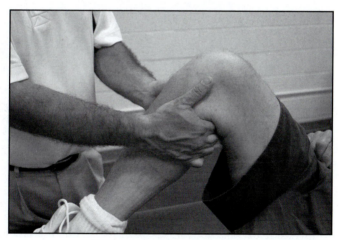

FIGURE 1-5. POPLITEAL PULSE.

CARDIOVASCULAR
SYSTEM

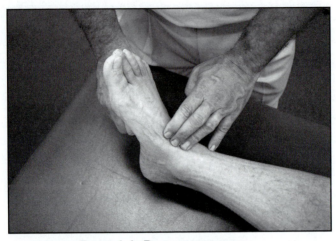

FIGURE 1-6. DORSALIS PEDIS PULSE.

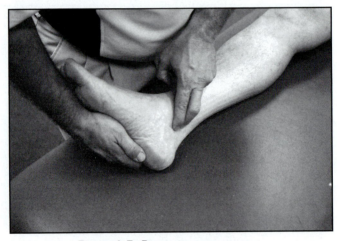

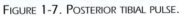

FIGURE 1-7. POSTERIOR TIBIAL PULSE.

BLOOD PRESSURE MEASUREMENT

TEST POSITION

- Supine with pillow under arm
- Seated, legs uncrossed, with fully exposed arm supported and relaxed at heart level so that the middle of the cuff is at the level of the right atrium (T4 or nipple)

ACTION

- Minimal 5-minute rest period
- Locate/mark brachial artery in antecubital fossa
- Place cuff around arm with mid-point of bladder in line with antecubital fossa head and cuff edge ~2 to 3 cm above and not touching stethoscope
- Bladder length = 80% and width = 40% of arm circumference in adults and children
- Locate/palpate radial pulse and inflate bladder >30 mm Hg above last palpable radial pulse
- Place bell of the stethoscope over artery
- Release pressure at ~2 to 3 mm/sec
- Record first and last audible sounds as the systolic and diastolic pressures

NORMAL FINDINGS[1]

- Healthy adults: systolic <120/ diastolic <80 mm Hg
  - ✧ Prehypertension 120-139/ or 80-89 mm Hg

POSITIVE FINDINGS

- Stage 1 hypertension = 140-159/ or 90-99[1]
- Stage 2 hypertension ≥160/ or ≥100[1]
- Auscultatory gap: a loss and then return of Korotkoff sounds due to venous engorgement of the upper extremity with poor antegrade flow[2]
  - ✧ More common in older, hypertensive clients with target organ damage[2]
- Pulsus paradoxus: >10 mm Hg fall in systolic pressure with inspiration is abnormal and a sign of pulmonary or pericardial disease but may be normal in obese or pregnant individuals[2]

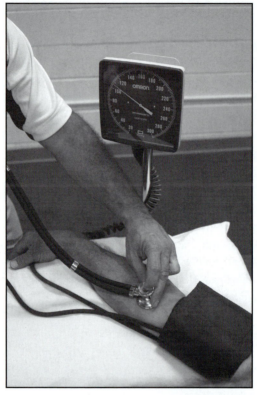

FIGURE 1-8. SUPINE BLOOD PRESSURE.

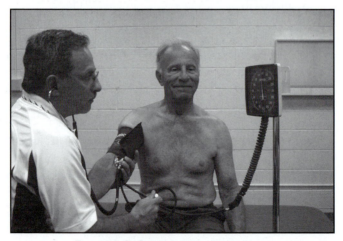

FIGURE 1-9. SITTING BLOOD PRESSURE.

Special Comments/Considerations[1]

- A mercury sphygmomanometer is preferred
- Measure both arms upon initial visit to detect coarctation of aorta and obstruction of upper extremity artery
- Right-to-left difference noted, record higher value
- Blood pressure can be measured bilaterally in women who are postmastectomy unless they have had lymphedema[1]
- Two readings should be obtained in each arm and averaged; rest at least 1 minute between readings
- Consecutive unilateral readings varying more than 5 mm Hg should be repeated and all readings should be averaged
- Evaluate further if bilateral findings vary >10 mm Hg
- Avoid assessing blood pressure immediately following exercise or alcohol or nicotine consumption
- In extremely obese clients, the cuff may be placed over the forearm and the appearance of radial pulse during deflation may be used as SBP
- For comfort, pregnant women may be measured in the left lateral recumbent position
- In suspected orthostatic hypotension, measure pressure in supine position, then again in seated or standing position
    - ✧ Decrease of >20 mm Hg suggests orthostatic hypotension[3]

References

1. Pickering TG, Hall JE, Appel LJ, et al. Recommendations for blood pressure measurement in humans and experimental animals: part 1: blood pressure measurements in humans: a statement for professionals from the subcommittee of professional and public education of the American Heart Association Council on High Blood Pressure Research. *Circulation.* 2005;111:697-716.

2. Chobanian AV, Bakris GL, Black HR, et al. Seventh report of the Joint National Committee on Prevention, Detection, Evaluation, and Treatment of High Blood Pressure. *Hypertension.* 2003;42:1206-1252.

3. Fang JC, O'Gara PT. Evaluation of the patient. In: Libby P, Bonow RO, Mann DL, Zipes DP, eds. *Braunwald's Heart Disease: A Textbook of Cardiovascular Medicine.* 8th ed. Philadelphia, PA: Saunders Co; 2008:131.

CARDIOVASCULAR
SYSTEM

PULSE PRESSURE

TEST POSITION (MEASUREMENT OVER BRACHIAL ARTERY)

- Supine with pillow under arm (maintain arm at heart level)
- Seated, legs uncrossed, supported, relaxed, fully exposed arm at heart level so that the mid cuff is at the level of the right atrium (T4 or nipple)

ACTION

- Locate/palpate radial pulse and inflate bladder >30 mm Hg above last palpable radial pulse
- Place bell of the stethoscope over artery
- Release pressure at ~2 to 3 mm/sec
- Record first and last audible sounds as the systolic and diastolic pressures
- Pulse pressure = Systolic pressure – Diastolic pressure[1]

NORMAL FINDINGS

- Pulse pressure increases with age[1,2]
- Values vary from an average of 30 to 50 mm Hg

POSITIVE FINDINGS

- Pulse pressure >60 mm Hg in older adults[3]
- Increased pulse pressure is predictive of congestive heart failure[4]

SPECIAL CONSIDERATIONS

- Low pulse pressure is a marker of low cardiac output in adults with acute heart failure[1]
- Increased pulse pressure indicates vascular wall (often aortic) stiffness[3] and predicts cardiovascular events independently, particularly heart failure in hypertensive clients[4]
- Increased pulse pressure can be found in aortic valve disorders, severe anemia, and overactive thyroid (hyperthyroidism)[3]
- Systolic and diastolic blood pressures are better predictors of mortality than pulse pressure[5]

REFERENCES

1. Terlink JR. Diagnosis and management of acute heart failure. In: Libby P, Bonow RO, Mann DL, Zipes DP, eds. *Braunwald's Heart Disease: A Textbook of Cardiovascular Medicine.* 8th ed. Philadelphia, PA: Saunders Co; 2008:583-610.

2. Pearson JD, Morrell CH, Brant LF, et al. Pulse pressure (systolic minus diastolic pressure with aging in apparently healthy subjects enrolled in the Baltimore Longitudinal Study of Aging. *J Gerontol Med Sci.* 1997;53:M177-183.

3. Mayo Clinics. http://www.mayoclinic.com/health/pulse-pressure/AN00968. Accessed March 18, 2010.

4. Haider AW, Larson MG, Franklin SS, Levy D. Systolic blood pressure, diastolic blood pressure, and pulse pressure as predictors of risk for congestive heart failure in the Framingham Heart Study. *Ann Intern Med.* 2003;138:10-16.

5. Pastor-Barriuso R, Banegas JR, Damián J, Appel LJ, Guallar E. Systolic blood pressure, diastolic blood pressure, and pulse pressure: an evaluation of their joint effect on mortality. *Ann Inter Med.* 2003;139:731-739.

RATE-PRESSURE PRODUCT OR DOUBLE PRODUCT

TEST POSITION
- Resting, seated upright with arm at heart level
- Also measured during upright exercise

ACTION
- Measure/record heart rate and systolic blood pressure (SBP)
- Rate-Pressure Product (RPP) = (heart rate [HR] x SBP) ÷ 100[1]

NORMAL FINDINGS
- RPP increases progressively during increasing exercise/work[2]

POSITIVE FINDINGS
- Large variation exists; a useful cut-off does not
- RPP does not progressively increase in those with significant ischemic heart disease[1]

SPECIAL CONSIDERATIONS
- RPP is an indirect method of estimating myocardial perfusion[2-4]
- Resting SBP and heart rate each vary by about 10 units and are generally lower than daytime measurements[2]
- Oxygen extraction in the coronary circulation is near maximal at rest; during exercise, perfusion MUST increase so that oxygen consumption demands are met[1]
- Perfusion increases only if heart rate increases and arteriolar resistance decreases[2]
- RPP is blunted in clients taking medications affecting heart rate

REFERENCES
1. Dwyer GB, Davis SE, ed. *ACSM's Health-Related Physical Fitness Assessment Manual.* 2nd ed. Philadelphia, PA: Lippincott Williams & Wilkins; 2008.
2. Libby P, Bonow RO, Mann DL, Zipes DP, eds. *Braunwald's Heart Disease: A Textbook of Cardiovascular Medicine.* 8th ed. Philadelphia, PA: Saunders Co; 2008.
3. Siegelova J, Fiser B, Dusek J, Placheta Z, Conrnelissen G, Halberg F. Circadian variability of rate-pressure product in essential hypertension with enalapril therapy. *Scripta medica (BRNO).* 2000;73:67-75.
4. Nelson RR, Gobel FL, Jorgensen CR, Wang K, Wang Y, Taylor HL. Hemodynamic predictors of myocardial oxygen consumption during static and dynamic exercise. *Circulation.* 1974;50:1179-1189.

ACUTE CHEST PAIN–CARDIAC ORIGIN

TEST POSITION

- Supine with bed at 30° elevation or any comfortable position for client

ACTION

- Obtain history of pain (duration, intensity, severity, aggravating, or relieving factors)
- Refer to Emergency Department based on history

NORMAL FINDINGS

- No chest pain
- Chest pain that can be reproduced over an affected costochondral joint, or reproduced with palpation, movement, or active resisted movements of the chest wall or arms is less likely to be of cardiac origin[1,2]

POSITIVE FINDINGS[1,2]

See Table 1-6 on the following page.

SPECIAL CONSIDERATION

- Duration, severity, and persistent symptoms unrelieved by rest should prompt referral

REFERENCES

1. Cannon CP, Lee TH. Approach to the patient with chest pain. In: Libby P, Bonow RO, Mann DL, Zipes DP, eds. *Braunwald's Heart Disease: A Textbook of Cardiovascular Medicine.* 8th ed. Philadelphia, PA: Saunders Co; 2008:1195-1205.
2. Newby LK, Douglas PS. Cardiovascular disease in women. In: Libby P, Bonow RO, Mann DL, Zipes DP, eds. *Braunwald's Heart Disease: A Textbook of Cardiovascular Medicine.* 8th ed. Philadelphia, PA: Saunders Co; 2008:1955-1966.

Table 1-6

CARDIAC CAUSES OF CHEST DISCOMFORT

Syndrome	Description	Key Features
Angina	Severe pressure, burning, or heaviness in the central-sternal region that may radiate to shoulders or left arm, neck, jaw, or epigastrium[1]; dyspnea; heartburn; abdominal pain; diaphoresis; dizziness[2]	May be precipitated by cold weather, work, exercise, or psychological stress[1] Duration <2-10 minutes[1]
Resting or unstable angina	Same as above, or more severe[1]	Typically <20 minutes; decreased exercise tolerance[1]
Acute myocardial infarction (men)	Same as above, or more severe[1]	Sudden onset, with duration of 30 minutes or longer Often accompanied by shortness of breath, weakness, nausea, vomiting[1]
Acute myocardial infarction (women)	May be same as above or milder[2] Chest pain may or may not be present Women without chest pain often report nausea/vomiting, indigestion, fatigue, sweating, arm/shoulder pain[2]	Symptoms described differently and may complain of prodromal fatigue[2]
Pericarditis	Sharp, pleuritic pain aggravated by changes in position[1]	Pericardial friction rub upon auscultation Variable duration of symptoms[1]

Adapted from Cannon CP, Lee TH. Approach to the patient with chest pain. In: Libby P, Bonow RO, Mann DL, Zipes DP, eds. *Braunwald's Heart Disease: A Textbook of Cardiovascular Medicine.* 8th ed. Philadelphia, PA: Saunders Co; 2008:1195-1205 and Newby LK, Douglas PS. Cardiovascular disease in women. In: Libby P, Bonow RO, Mann DL, Zipes DP, eds. *Braunwald's Heart Disease: A Textbook of Cardiovascular Medicine.* 8th ed. Philadelphia, PA: Saunders Co; 2008:1955-1966.

ANGINA PAIN RATING SCALE

TEST POSITION

- Any position during or following activity

ACTION

- Show and explain scale
- Client identifies angina level

NORMAL FINDINGS

- No report of angina

POSITIVE FINDINGS

- Burning, crushing, strangling, constricting, suffocating, squeezing pressure in chest[1]

Table 1-7

RATING OF CHEST DISCOMFORT

Rating	Nonexercise Conditions[2]	Exercise Conditions[3]
1	Mild, barely noticeable discomfort	Mild, typical angina
2	Moderate, bothersome	Moderate to severe, tolerable
3	Severe, very uncomfortable	Severe, exercise often stopped by client
4	Extremely severe, unbearable	Extremely severe, unbearable

Adapted from Rothstein JM, Roy SH, Wolf SL. *The Rehabilitation Specialist's Handbook*. 3rd ed. Philadelphia, PA: F.A. Davis; 2005, and Fletcher GF, Balady GJ, Amsterdam EA, et al. Exercise standards for testing and training: a statement for healthcare professionals from the American Heart Association. *Circulation*. 2001;104:1694-1740.

SPECIAL CONSIDERATIONS

- Clients should be seated prior to taking medication as it may lead to peripheral vasodilatation
- Clients with known angina should carry nitroglycerin and take as prescribed

CARDIOVASCULAR
SYSTEM

- Unrelieved angina following rest or nitroglycerin protocol requires activation of emergency medical services (EMS)
- Cases in which angina is perceived as different from typical, occurs at rest, or increased in frequency and severity should be reported immediately to primary health care provider
- Characteristics of nonischemic chest pain include a) localized to the tip of one finger, b) reproduced during palpation or a manual muscle test, c) duration of a few seconds or many hours, d) does not radiate to lower extremities, e) a sharp pain associated with coughing or chest movement[1]

REFERENCES

1. Cannon CP, Lee TH. Approach to the patient with chest pain. In: Libby P, Bonow RO, Mann DL, Zipes DP, eds. *Braunwald's Heart Disease: A Textbook of Cardiovascular Medicine*. 8th ed. Philadelphia, PA: Saunders Co; 2008:1195-1206.
2. Rothstein JM, Roy SH, Wolf SL. *The Rehabilitation Specialist's Handbook*. 3rd ed. Philadelphia, PA: F.A. Davis; 2005.
3. Fletcher GF, Balady GJ, Amsterdam EA, et al. Exercise standards for testing and training: a statement for healthcare professionals from the American Heart Association. *Circulation*. 2001;104:1694-1740.

OTHER SOURCES OF CHEST PAIN

TEST POSITION

- Supine or with bed at 30° elevation

ACTION

- History and palpation

NORMAL FINDINGS

- Infrequent, fleeting pains/aches or soreness related to muscular work

POSITIVE FINDINGS

- Acute pericarditis usually causes fever and chest pain typically extending to the left shoulder and/or down the left arm
  - ◇ Pain may be similar to that of a heart attack, but it tends to be made worse by lying down, swallowing food, coughing, or even deep breathing

See Table 1-8 on the following pages.

SPECIAL CONSIDERATION

- Table 1-8 is not all inclusive; any client reporting acute chest pain should be carefully examined and referred to emergent care or the proper specialist for further evaluation.

Table 1-8

OTHER CAUSES OF CHEST DISCOMFORT

Category	Possible Etiology	Relieving Factors	Other
Esophageal disorders	Reflux, diffuse spasms with vigorous to high-amplitude peristaltic contractions, achalasia[1]	Nitroglycerin, antacids, warm liquids, milk, or food	Esophageal and cardiac disorders can coexist[1]
Biliary colic	Gall bladder, liver, and bile duct disorders[1]	Spontaneous pain relief[1]	Asymptomatic between attacks, which generally consist of steady pain, lasting 2-4 hours Pain most intense in right upper abdominal quadrant Precordial or epigastric pain possible Pain may be referred to scapula, posterior costal margins, and, rarely, to the shoulder[1]
Costosternal syndrome	Inflamed costal cartilage,[1] often at 4th, 5th, and 6th ribs	Rest, anti-inflammatory medications, physical therapy	Localized and frequently reproduced upon palpation Myocardial etiology must be ruled out

(continued)

Table 1-8 (continued)

OTHER CAUSES OF CHEST DISCOMFORT

Category	Possible Etiology	Relieving Factors	Other
Other musculoskeletal disorders	Cervical radiculitis, bursitis, arthritis, brachial plexus compression, left shoulder tendonitis	Physical therapy, osteopathy	Constant ache, sometimes sensory deficit noted[1] Discerned through careful musculoskeletal screening
Acute myocardial infarction	Coronary occlusion	None, emergent care required	Prolonged intense pain (>30 minutes)[2] Associated with nausea, vomiting, diaphoresis, dyspnea, weakness[2]
Aortic dissection	Tearing of aortic intimal lining via trauma, atherosclerosis, or hypertension	Emergent care required	Described as a excruciating "tearing" or "ripping" chest pain that may radiate posteriorly[2] True medical emergency
Pulmonary hypertension	Unknown, familial, congenital, connective tissue diseases, left-sided heart or valve disease, lung disease and/or hypoxemia, chronic thrombotic or embolic disease, sickle-cell, as well as numerous other causes[3]	Treating underlying heart or lung disease, supplemental oxygen, digoxin, calcium-channel blockers, diuretics, vasodilators, endothelin receptor antagonists, lung transplantation[3]	Substernal chest pain[2] with dyspnea Right ventricular failure (cor pulmonale) or failure with exercise is a possible outcome[3] Syncope, paroxysmal nocturnal dyspnea, orthopnea are all possible outcomes[3]

(continued)

Table 1-8 (continued)

OTHER CAUSES OF CHEST DISCOMFORT

Category	Possible Etiology	Relieving Factors	Other
Pulmonary embolism	Venous stasis, hypercoagulability, wall trauma[4]	Oxygenation/mechanical ventilation, anticoagulant therapy	Cardinal symptoms: dyspnea and tachypnea Dyspnea, syncope, cyanosis without chest pain represent life-threatening signs[4]
Pleuritic pain	Pleural inflammation, fluid accumulation (effusion), pneumothorax (air or gas build-up), hemothorax (blood accumulation)	Splinting, thoracentesis, medical treatment of underlying condition, pain medication	Sharp, knife-like pain or coughing, cyanosis, dyspnea, tachypnea, and, in some cases, pleural friction rub
Acute pericarditis	Swelling and irritation of pericardium most often due to unknown causes (viral etiology)	Pain management, treating underlying etiology	Cardinal sign: chest pain unrelieved by rest or nitroglycerin Pericardial friction rub at left lower sternal border[5] Chest pain worsens with inspiration, movement, swallowing, and supine positioning; improves with forward sitting[5]

REFERENCES

1. Morrow DA, Gersh BJ. Chronic coronary artery disease. In: Libby P, Bonow RO, Mann DL, Zipes DP, eds. *Braunwald's Heart Disease: A Textbook of Cardiovascular Medicine.* 8th ed. Philadelphia, PA: Saunders Co; 2008:1354.

2. Cannon CP, Lee TH. Approach to the patient with chest pain. In: Libby P, Bonow RO, Mann DL, Zipes DP, eds. *Braunwald's Heart Disease: A Textbook of Cardiovascular Medicine.* 8th ed. Philadelphia, PA: Saunders Co; 2008:1195-1205.

3. Rich S, McLaughlin VV. Pulmonary hypertension. In: Libby P, Bonow RO, Mann DL, Zipes DP, eds. *Braunwald's Heart Disease: A Textbook of Cardiovascular Medicine.* 8th ed. Philadelphia, PA: Saunders Co; 2008:1883-1914.

4. Goldhaber SA. Pulmonary embolism. In: Libby P, Bonow RO, Mann DL, Zipes DP, eds. *Braunwald's Heart Disease: A Textbook of Cardiovascular Medicine.* 8th ed. Philadelphia, PA: Saunders Co; 2008:1863-1882.

5. LeWinter MM. Pericardial diseases. In: Libby P, Bonow RO, Mann DL, Zipes DP, eds. *Braunwald's Heart Disease: A Textbook of Cardiovascular Medicine.* 8th ed. Philadelphia, PA: Saunders Co; 2008:1829-1854.

CARDIAC INSPECTION AND PALPATION

TEST POSITION
- Supine with bed at 30° elevation, head on small pillow
- Left lateral decubitus (side lying) or forward sitting position if apical impulse not detected when supine[1]

ACTION
- Stand on right and inspect entire anterior thorax for scars and pulsations
- Using tangential light, inspect anterior chest for apical impulse or point of maximal impulse[1]

Table 1-9

CARDIAC PALPATION SITES

Palpation Location[1]	Structure[1]
2nd right intercostal space (ICS)	Aortic area
2nd left ICS	Pulmonary area
3rd-5th ICS, left sternal border or in epigastric or subxiphoid area	Right ventricular area
4th-5th left ICS at or medial to midclavicular line	Left ventricular area

Adapted from Bickley LS. *Bates' Pocket Guide to Physical Examination and History Taking*. 10th ed. Philadelphia, PA: Lippincott Williams & Wilkins; 2009.

PALPATION
- Palpate all areas in order with pads of fingers, followed by heel of hand[1]
  - ❖ Finger pad palpation best detects heaves or lifts[1]—ventricular impulses lifting palpating fingers[1]
  - ❖ Heel of hand best reveals thrills[1]—vibratory sensations always felt with murmurs[2]
  - ❖ Palpate apical impulse and/or point of maximal impulse (PMI) with one finger and note location, diameter, amplitude, duration; palpate apical impulse in supine or left lateral position

NORMAL FINDINGS

- Healed scars, no heaves, lifts, or thrills[1]
- Visible apical pulsation in young, thin, or those with nonmuscular chest walls
- Apical impulse location (4th or 5th ICS from xiphoid to left midclavicular line), diameter (<2.5 cm), amplitude (small, feels brisk-like tapping), duration (< 2/3 of S1)[1]
- Apical impulse is often the PMI[1]

POSITIVE FINDINGS

- Visible pulsations other than apical,[3] heaves, lifts, or thrills[1]
- Apical impulse is not point of maximal impulse

SPECIAL CONSIDERATIONS

- Exhalation, then breath holding may help during palpation[1]
- Apical impulse is the early pulsation of the left ventricle as it touches the chest wall during contraction and only palpable in about half of adults[1]
- Apical impulse and point of maximal impulse are usually same location; if different, pathology[1] should be considered
- Heaves or lifts: Large cardiac pulsations upon palpation associated with ventricular hypertrophy[4]
- Thrill: Vibratory sensation associated with murmurs (feels like a purring cat's neck) and is felt on the body surface[2]

REFERENCES

1. Bickley LS. *Bates' Pocket Guide to Physical Examination and History Taking.* 10th ed. Philadelphia, PA: Lippincott Williams & Wilkins; 2009.
2. The Cardiac Exam: Palpation. http://filer.case.edu/~dck3/heart/palpate.html. Accessed March 18, 2010.
3. Fang JC, O'Gara PT. The history and physical examination: an evidence-based approach. In: Libby P, Bonow RO, Mann DL, Zipes DP, eds. *Braunwald's Heart Disease: A Textbook of Cardiovascular Medicine.* 8th ed. Philadelphia, PA: Saunders Co; 2008:125-148.
4. Jarvis C. *Physical Examination and Health Assessment.* 5th ed. St. Louis, MO: Saunders-Elsevier; 2008.

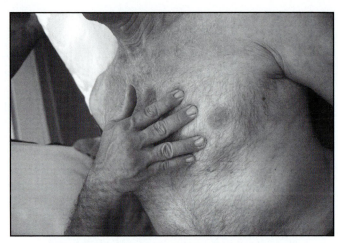

FIGURE 1-10. FINGERPAD PALPATION.

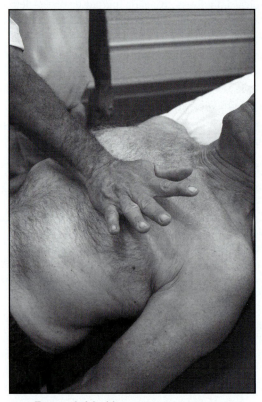

FIGURE 1-11. HEEL OF HAND PALPATION.

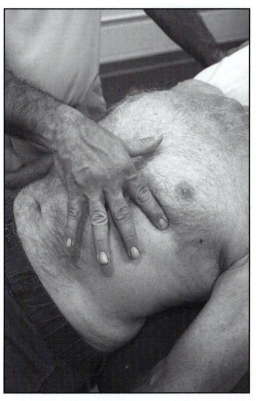

FIGURE 1-12. APICAL IMPULSE PALPATION.

AUSCULTATION

TEST POSITION[1]

- 1st: Supine with bed at 30° elevation, head on small pillow
  - ✧ Use stethoscope diaphragm in all areas
  - ✧ Attend to tricuspid area with bell of stethoscope
- 2nd: Left lateral decubitus position,[1] particularly for S3
  - ✧ Attend to apex with stethoscope bell
- 3rd: Seated position, forward lean, exhalation, hold breath
  - ✧ Attend to left sternal border and apex with diaphragm

ACTION[1]

- Complete inspection and palpation, then auscultate
- Stand on client's right side
- With stethoscope diaphragm (firm pressure), then bell (light pressure), auscultate over aortic, pulmonic, tricuspid, and apex/mitral valve areas
- Diaphragm: High-pitched sounds, S1, S2, aortic/mitral regurgitation, pericardial friction rubs
- Bell: Low-pitched sounds, S3, S4, mitral stenosis murmur

Table 1-10

CARDIAC AUSCULTATION SITES

2nd right intercostal space (ICS)	Aortic valve area
2nd-3rd left ICS	Pulmonic valve area
4th-5th left ICS	Tricuspid valve area
4th-5th ICS at or medial to midclavicular line	Apical/mitral valve area

NORMAL FINDINGS[1]

- High-pitched sounds best heard with diaphragm of stethoscope
- S1 is heard best at apex, S2 heard best at base[1]

Table 1-11

NORMAL HEART SOUNDS

Name	Sounds Like	Closing Of	Systole
S1	Lub	Mitral, tricuspid valves	Begins
S2	Dub	Aortic, pulmonic valves	Ends

Adapted from Bickley LS, Szilagyi PG. *Bates' Guide to Physical Examination and History Taking.* 9th ed. Philadelphia, PA: Lippincott Williams & Wilkins; 2007.

POSITIVE FINDINGS[1]

- Low-pitched sounds best heard with bell of stethoscope
- May be heard with light pressure and not heard with alternating firm pressure
- Variations in S1 or S2
- Extra sounds in systole or diastole
- Murmurs: Pansystolic (holosystolic), midsystolic, pathologic, diastolic murmurs, sounds with systolic and diastolic components[1]

Table 1-12

S3 AND S4 HEART SOUNDS

Name	Sounds Like	May Suggest
S3	Lub dub dee	Heart failure, diastolic dysfunction[2]
S4	Dee lub dub	Noncompliant or hypertrophic ventricle[3]
S3 or S4	---	Either sound is normal in athletes[1]

CARDIOVASCULAR SYSTEM

SPECIAL CONSIDERATIONS

- Use quality stethoscope with short hose (take up slack), diaphragm held against skin
- S3 may be normal up to age 40 and during last trimester of pregnancy
- S3, when pathologic, is known as a ventricular gallop
- S4 occurs in late diastole and is known as an atrial gallop
- Murmurs are described by timing, shape, location, radiation, and intensity[1]
- Broad categories of abnormalities are listed here. Readers should review appropriate audio material and work with an experienced mentor

REFERENCES

1. Bickley LS, Szilagyi PG. *Bates' Guide to Physical Examination and History Taking.* 9th ed. Philadelphia, PA: Lippincott Williams & Wilkins; 2007.
2. Fang JC, O'Gara PT. The history and physical examination: an evidence-based approach. In: Libby P, Bonow RO, Mann DL, Zipes DP, eds. *Braunwald's Heart Disease: A Textbook of Cardiovascular Medicine.* 8th ed. Philadelphia, PA: Saunders Co; 2008:134.
3. Jarvis C. *Physical Examination and Health Assessment.* 5th ed. St. Louis, MO: Saunders-Elsevier; 2008.

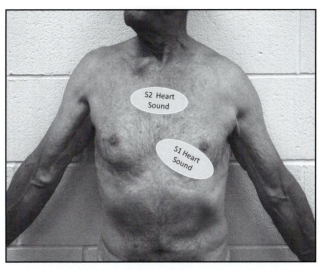

FIGURE 1-13. S1 AND S2 HEART SOUNDS.

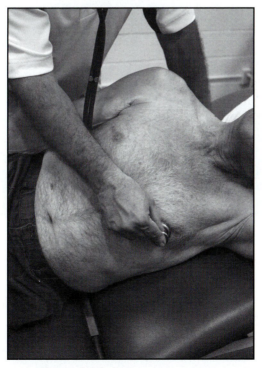

FIGURE 1-14. LEFT LATERAL POSITION.

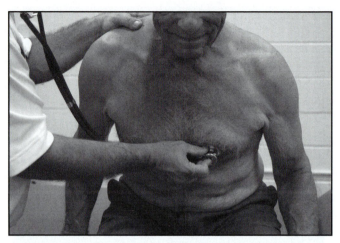

FIGURE 1-15. SEATED POSITION.

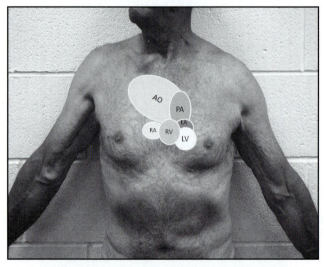

FIGURE 1-16. AREAS OF AUSCULTATION.

JUGULAR VENOUS DISTENSION

TEST POSITION
- Supine with bed at 30° elevation, head on small pillow
- Head turned slightly away from clinician

ACTION
- Shine light obliquely on neck to locate jugular pulsations
- Internal jugular vein is deep within the sternocleidomastoid muscle
- Place vertical ruler atop the manubriosternal junction
- Place second ruler perpendicular to first ruler
- Measure height of jugular venous pulsation in centimeters

NORMAL FINDINGS
- Venous column <3 cm above the manubriosternal junction

POSITIVE FINDINGS
- Venous column 3 to 5 cm above the manubriosternal junction

SPECIAL CONSIDERATIONS
- Internal jugular vein is medial to external jugular vein and extends on an approximate line from the earlobe to the sternoclavicular joint
- Jugular venous pressure reflects left ventricular filling pressure[1]
- Jugular venous distension is predictive for heart failure hospitalizations and heart failure death[1]
- Use external jugular vein if internal jugular vein is difficult to locate[2]

REFERENCES
1. Fang JC, O'Gara PT. The history and physical examination: an evidence-based approach. In: Libby P, Bonow RO, Mann DL, Zipes DP, eds. *Braunwald's Heart Disease: A Textbook of Cardiovascular Medicine.* 8th ed. Philadelphia, PA: Saunders Co; 2008:134.
2. Bickley LS, Szilagyi PG. *Bates' Guide to Physical Examination and History Taking.* 9th ed. Philadelphia, PA: Lippincott Williams & Wilkins; 2007.

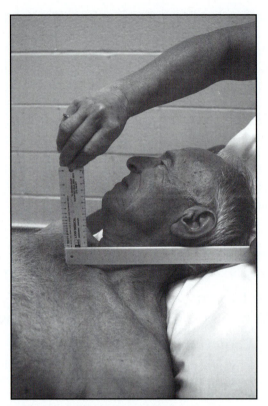

FIGURE 1-17. JUGULAR VENOUS DISTENSION.

Section

Two

Examination of the
Pulmonary System

PULMONARY
SYSTEM

RESPIRATORY HISTORY

Do you have any discomfort or uncomfortable feelings in your chest?[1]

Table 2-1

QUESTIONS RELATED TO PULMONARY COMPLAINTS[1,2]

O nset	When did it first occur? Gradual or sudden?
L ocation	Can you point to the specific location?
D uration	How long does the discomfort last?
C haracter	Can you describe the discomfort? If painful, how bad is it on a scale of 1-10?
A ggravating/ **A** lleviating factors	What makes it better? What makes it worse?
R adiation	Does the discomfort radiate or move?
T iming	Is the discomfort always there or does it come and go? Is it related to anything?
S igns or symptoms	Any other signs or symptoms that occur with the discomfort?

Adapted from Bickley LS, Szilagyi PG. *Bates' Guide to Physical Examination and History Taking.* 9th ed. Philadelphia, PA: Lippincott Williams & Wilkins; 2007.

REFERENCES

1. Bickley LS, Szilagyi PG. *Bates' Guide to Physical Examination and History Taking.* 9th ed. Philadelphia, PA: Lippincott Williams & Wilkins; 2007.

2. Jarvis C. *Physical Examination and Health Assessment.* 5th ed. St. Louis, MO: Saunders-Elsevier; 2008.

Table 2-2

SIGNS AND SYMPTOMS OF RESPIRATORY DISTRESS[1,2]

Sign/ Symptom	Possible Pulmonary Pathology	Be Sure to Ask About	Other Possible Pathologies
Cough	Acute or chronically irritated receptors within large airways due to bacterial or viral agents, inflammation, increased pressure, increased tension	• Is your cough wet or dry?[2] • If wet, how much (volume, give examples: tsp, tbsp, shot glass, cup) • What is the color?[2]	Left heart failure or mitral stenosis, pulmonary embolism, irritating inhalants, lung neoplasm
Chest pain	Tracheobronchitis, pleuritic pain[1]	• Does it feel like a squeezing, heavy pressure? • How long does it last? • Does it go away with rest or medication? • Does it feel like ripping or tearing?	Angina, myocardial infarction, pericarditis, dissecting aneurysm, reflux esophagitis or esophageal spasm, costochondritic pain, musculotendinous pain, anxiety, arthritis[1]
Dyspnea	Chronic bronchitis or emphysema, asthma, various interstitial diseases (sarcoidosis, asbestosis, pulmonary fibrosis, cancer), pneumonia, pneumothorax, acute embolism, and anxiety causing hyperventilation	• How much activity (walking distance, stair-climbing, vacuuming, etc) can you do before you need to slow down or stop?	Heart failure, valvular disease

(continued)

PULMONARY
SYSTEM

Table 2-2 (continued)

SIGNS AND SYMPTOMS OF RESPIRATORY DISTRESS[1,2]

Sign/Symptom	Possible Pulmonary Pathology	Be Sure to Ask About	Other Possible Pathologies
Hemoptysis	Bacterial pneumonia, chronic bronchitis, bronchiectasis, tuberculosis, abscess, neoplasm, pulmonary emboli	• OLD CAARTS (see Table 2-1)	Heart failure or mitral stenosis
Wheezing	Narrowed airways due to smooth muscle constriction or mucus accumulation	• Are you ok?	Smooth muscle constriction can be due to emphysema, irritants, exercise, cold air

Adapted from Bickley LS, Szilagyi PG. *Bates' Guide to Physical Examination and History Taking.* 9th ed. Philadelphia, PA: Lippincott Williams & Wilkins; 2007.

INSPECTION OF THE THORAX

TEST POSITION
- Seated for posterior thorax; seated/supine for anterior thorax

ACTION
- Observe posterior, then anterior thorax for shape, coloration, scars, skin lesions, intercostal retractions, abnormal movements, or muscle contractions

NORMAL FINDINGS
- Midline trachea
- Symmetrical chest, actively and uniformly moving upward and forward during inspiration and passively inward and downward during expiration
- Approximately a 2:1 anterior-posterior diameter

POSITIVE FINDINGS
- Use BAD CAT mnemonic

Table 2-3

BAD CAT—ALARMING RESPIRATORY SIGNS

B	A	D	C	A	T
Breathing that is audible	Active accessory muscles	Dyspnea	Cyanosis or clubbing	Anterior posterior diameter ≥ 1.0	Tracheal deviation from midline

---

- Posterior interspace or supraclavicular retraction with inspiration
- Anterior lower interspace retraction with inspiration
- Impaired unilateral or bilateral movement or delay
- Asymmetrical thorax shape, including: kyphosis, scoliosis, barrel chest, pectus excavatum, and pectus carinatum

SPECIAL CONSIDERATIONS
- Structural abnormalities may limit thorax and lung compliance

PULMONARY SYSTEM

- Structural abnormalities or lung disease may lead to dyspnea
  - ✧ Kyphosis: An accentuated thoracic curve appearing as a "hump"
  - ✧ Scoliosis: A shift of the spinous processes from the midline, forming a curve to the right or left within the frontal plane
  - ✧ Barrel chest: A condition where the depth of anterior-posterior thorax approaches the thorax width
  - ✧ Pectus excavatum: A congenital defect where the sternum appears sunken[2,3]
  - ✧ Pectus carinatum: A congenital defect where the sternum is raised; "pigeon chest"[2,3]
- Those with dyspnea often self-select positions of comfort

REFERENCES

1. Bickley LS, Szilagyi PG. *Bates' Guide to Physical Examination and History Taking.* 9th ed. Philadelphia, PA: Lippincott Williams & Wilkins; 2007.
2. What is pectus excavatum/carinatum? http://www.pectus.org/whatis.htm. Accessed March 18, 2010.
3. UK Pectus Excavatum and Pectus Carinatum Information Site. http://www.pectus.org/contacts.htm. Accessed March 18, 2010.

PULMONARY SYSTEM

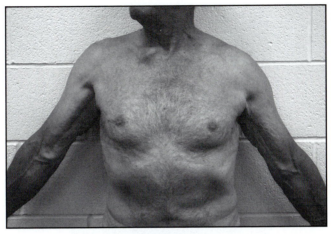

FIGURE 2-1. ANTERIOR.

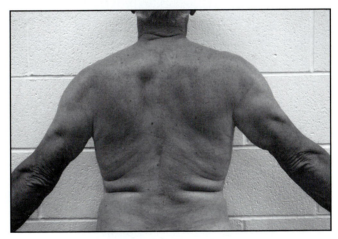

FIGURE 2-2. POSTERIOR.

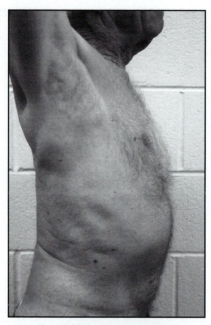

FIGURE 2-3. RIGHT LATERAL.

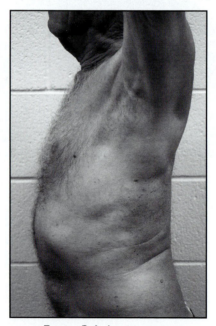

FIGURE 2-4. LEFT LATERAL.

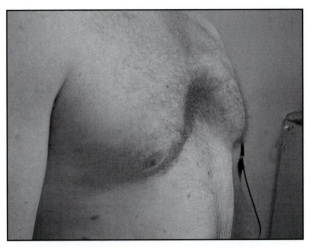

FIGURE 2-5. PECTUS EXCAVATUM.

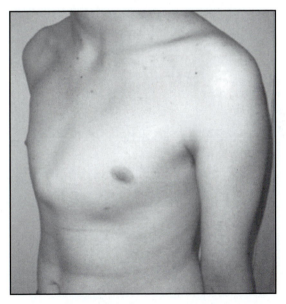

FIGURE 2-6. PECTUS CARINATUM.

PULMONARY
SYSTEM

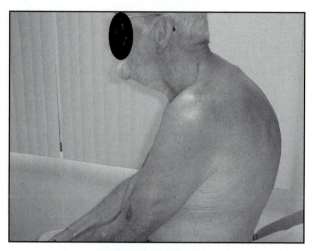

FIGURE 2-7. KYPHOSIS.

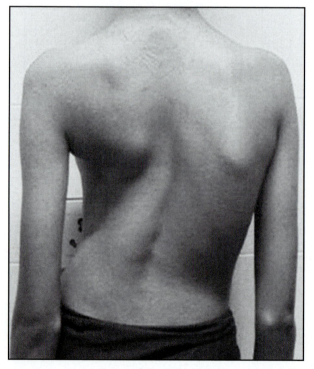

FIGURE 2-8. SCOLIOSIS.

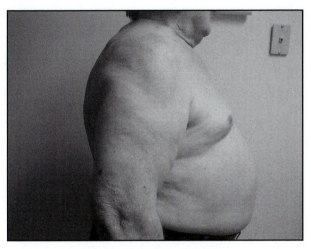

FIGURE 2-9. BARREL CHEST.

PULMONARY ANATOMY

LEFT LUNG
- Has upper and lower lobes

RIGHT LUNG
- Has an upper, lower, and middle lobe

GROSS ANATOMY
- Posterior
  - ✧ Superior border is ~T3/T4
  - ✧ Inferior border is ~T10 and descends further with inspiration
  - ✧ Vertical lines along spinous processes and inferior angle of scapula
- Anterior
  - ✧ Apices rise ~2-4 cm above the medial third of clavicle
  - ✧ Lower medial border is at ~6th rib, lateral border ~8th rib
- Lateral
  - ✧ Vertical lines just anterior and posterior to the deltoid form axillary lines
  - ✧ Midaxillary line: a third axillary line running beneath the deltoid, halfway between the anterior and posterior axillary lines
- Oblique fissures divide lungs into oblique anterior and posterior halves from ~T3 spinous process to ~ anterior 6th intercostal space at the midclavicular line
- Horizontal fissure divides anterior portion of right lung into upper and middle lobes

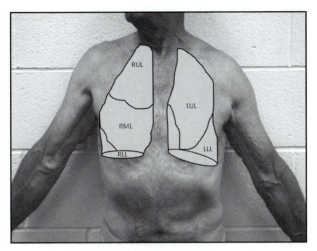

FIGURE 2-10. ANTERIOR.

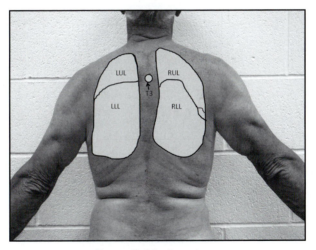

FIGURE 2-11. POSTERIOR.

PULMONARY
SYSTEM

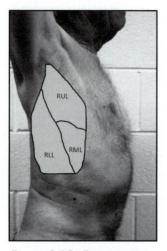

FIGURE 2-12. RIGHT LATERAL.

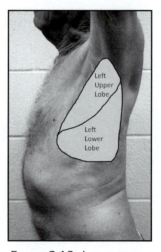

FIGURE 2-13. LEFT LATERAL.

RESPIRATORY RATE

TEST POSITION

- Seated, supine, or side lying

ACTION

- Pretend to be assessing radial pulse, observe/count respirations[1]
- Alternatively, place stethoscope bell over upper sternum[1]
- Count the number of breaths in 15 seconds, multiply by 4[1]
- Note respiratory rhythm; if irregular, count breaths for 30 to 60 seconds[1]
- Normal rate should allow for normal tidal volume

NORMAL FINDINGS[2]

Table 2-4

BREATHING FREQUENCY

Age	Breaths per minute
Neonate	30-40
1-2	20-40
3-10	20-30
11-15	18-22
16-Adult	12-20

Adapted from Jarvis C. *Physical Examination and Health Assessment.* 5th ed. St. Louis, MO: Saunders-Elsevier; 2008.

POSITIVE FINDINGS

- Bradypnea: Respiratory rate ≤10 per minute in adults[1]
  - ✧ Tidal volume may be normal
- Tachypnea: Respiratory rate ≥22 per minute in adults[1]
- Tidal volume will likely be low

SPECIAL CONSIDERATIONS

- Preserve modesty via draping
- Avoid making obvious respiratory rate measurement
- Careful monitoring of tidal volume and rhythm

REFERENCES

1. Wilms JL, Schneiderman H, Algranati PS. *Physical Diagnosis: Bedside Evaluation of Diagnosis and Function.* Baltimore, MD: Williams & Wilkins; 1994.
2. Jarvis C. *Physical Examination and Health Assessment.* 5th ed. St. Louis, MO: Saunders-Elsevier; 2008.

PULMONARY SYSTEM

RESPIRATORY RHYTHM

TEST POSITION
- Seated

ACTION
- Pretend to be assessing radial pulse, observe/count respirations[1]
- Alternatively, place stethoscope bell over upper sternum[1]
- Note respiratory rhythm; if irregular, count breaths for 30 to 60 seconds[1]

NORMAL FINDINGS
- Expiration approximately 2 times longer than inspiration[1]
- Sighing can be a normal phenomenon with tidal volumes 2 to 3 times greater than normal
- Adult sigh rate: 9 to 10 per hour[2]
- Infant sigh rate: 18 to 70 per hour during the first 24 hours of life[2]; 6 to 36 per hour at the 5th day of life[2]
- Sighs may occur during inspiration or expiration[2]

POSITIVE FINDINGS
- Apnea: Long delay between breaths
- Biot's: Irregular cycles of uniformly deep or shallow breaths separated by apnea
  - ✧ Seen with lower pontine and medullary disorders, meningitis, posterior fossa lesions, morphine poisoning, hypercapnic stupor[3]
- Cheyne-Stokes: Long periods of regularly alternating phases of hyperventilation and apnea due to cerebral embolism, cerebral infarction, lactic acidosis, diabetic ketoacidosis, uremic coma[3]
  - ✧ Periodic breathing: A form of Cheyne-Stokes respiration where tidal volume varies for periods by more than half
- Kussmaul breathing: A form of hyperventilation with increased depth (often labored), normal, or abnormal rate[4]
  - ✧ Seen in those with severe acidosis[1]
- Obstructive breathing: Normal inspiration but prolonged expiration

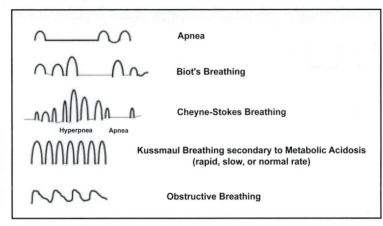

FIGURE 2-14. APNEA, BIOT'S BREATHING, CHEYNE-STOKES BREATHING, KUSSMAUL BREATHING, OBSTRUCTIVE BREATHING.

SPECIAL CONSIDERATION
- Avoid obvious measurement of respiratory rhythm

REFERENCES
1. Finesilver C. Pulmonary assessment: what you need to know. *Prog Cardiovasc Nurs.* 2003;18:83-92.

2. Sighing. http://www.answers.com/topic/sighing?cat=health. Accessed March 19, 2010.

3. Prakash UBS, King TE. Neurologic diseases. In: Crapo JD, Glassroth J, Karlinsky JB, King TE, eds. *Baum's Textbook of Pulmonary Diseases.* 7th ed. Philadelphia, PA: Lippincott Williams & Wilkins; 2004.

4. Wilms JL, Schneiderman H, Algranati PS. *Physical Diagnosis: Bedside Evaluation of Diagnosis and Function.* Baltimore, MD: Williams & Wilkins; 1994.

PULMONARY SYSTEM

RESPIRATORY DEPTH AND SYMMETRY OF MOVEMENT

TEST POSITION

- Seated

ACTION

- Lightly place hands over chest, thumb tips slightly apart, free to move
- Palms should draw skin medially prior to deep inspiration
- Upper lobes: Place palms atop clavicles, fingers extended superiorly over trapezius, thumbs at sternoclavicular joints[1]
- Right middle lobe and left lingual lobe: Place fingers anterolaterally at posterior axillary folds[1]
- Lower lobes: Place thumbs at T9,10 spinous process[2]
- Estimate chest expansion by distance thumbs move during inspiration

NORMAL FINDINGS

- Symmetric, 3 to 5 cm expansion

POSITIVE FINDINGS

- Less than 3-cm movement
- Unilateral delay suggests atelectasis, pneumonia, and postoperative guarding[2]

SPECIAL CONSIDERATION

- Privacy and appropriate draping

REFERENCES

1. Hillegas EA, Sadowsky SH. *Essentials of Cardiopulmonary Physical Therapy.* 2nd ed. Philadelphia, PA: WB Saunders Co; 2006:631.
2. Jarvis C. *Physical Examination and Health Assessment.* 5th ed. St. Louis, MO: Saunders-Elsevier; 2008.

PULMONARY SYSTEM

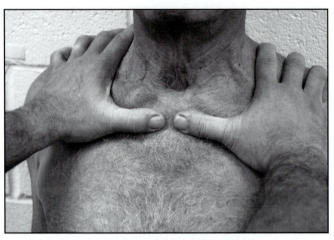

FIGURE 2-15. UPPER LOBES (REST).

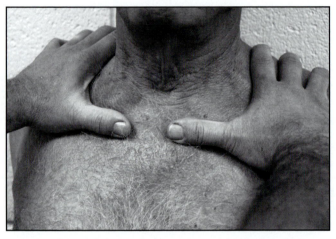

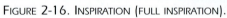

FIGURE 2-16. INSPIRATION (FULL INSPIRATION).

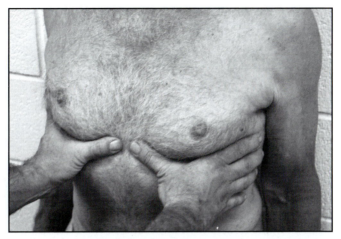

FIGURE 2-17. RIGHT MIDDLE LOBE AND LEFT LINGUAL LOBE (REST).

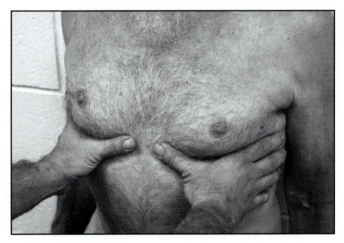

FIGURE 2-18. RIGHT MIDDLE LOBE AND LEFT LINGUAL LOBE
(FULL INSPIRATION).

PULMONARY
SYSTEM

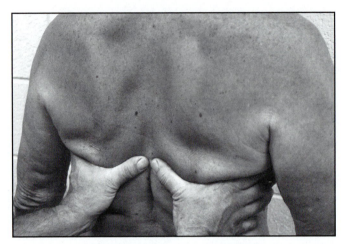

FIGURE 2-19. LOWER LOBES (REST).

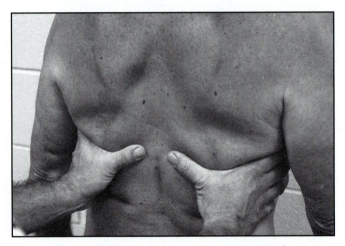

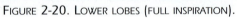

FIGURE 2-20. LOWER LOBES (FULL INSPIRATION).

THORACIC DEPTH, WIDTH, AND DIAMETER

TEST POSITION

- Standing

ACTION

- Large spreading caliper at T4 xiphisternal line (~nipple level) for chest depth and width
- Measure at full inspiration and full expiration and use means for calculation[1]

NORMAL FINDINGS

- Barrel chest normally seen in infancy and often with aging
- Young and middle-age adults, anterior-posterior (AP) diameter is ~½ of transverse diameter[2]
- Chest expansion via caliper in healthy youths, adults, and older adults is similar in width and depth[3]
- Average transverse diameter measured via caliper is slightly greater than AP diameter[3]

See Table 2-5 on the following page.

POSITIVE FINDINGS

- Barrel chest: AP diameter ≥ transverse diameter (≥1:1 ratio)
- Barrel chest commonly reported as sign of chronic obstructive lung disease[2]

SPECIAL CONSIDERATIONS

- Mean values may be significantly greater in those with chronic obstructive pulmonary disease (COPD), ranges overlap[1]
- Changes may be a function of aging, rather than disease[1]
- Inter- and intrarater reliabilities $>r = 0.963$[1]

REFERENCES

1. Klipstein-Grobusch K, Georg T, Boeing H. Interviewer variability in anthropometric measurements and estimates of body composition. *Int J Epidemiol.* 1997;26:S174-S180.

2. Bickley LS, Szilagyi PG. *Bates' Guide to Physical Examination and History Taking.* 9th ed. Philadelphia, PA: Lippincott Williams & Wilkins; 2007.

3. Moll JM, Wright V. An objective clinical study of chest expansion. *Ann Rheum Dis.* 1972;31:1-8.

PULMONARY SYSTEM

PULMONARY SYSTEM

Table 2-5

Average Changes in Thoracic Transverse and Anterior-Posterior Diameter in Healthy Adolescents, Adults, and Older Adults

Age (yrs)	15-24	15-24	25-34	25-34	35-44	35-44	45-54	45-54	55-64	55-64	65-74	65-74	75+	75+
Gender	♂	♀	♂	♀	♂	♀	♂	♀	♂	♀	♂	♀	♂	♀
Transverse	2.64	2.3	2.98	2.66	2.96	2.41	2.58	2.33	2.27	1.83	1.73	1.85	1.47	.96
AP	2.54	2.13	3.17	2.08	2.50	1.77	2.34	1.94	2.17	1.75	1.61	1.53	1.78	1.40

Adapted from Moll JM, Wright V. An objective clinical study of chest expansion. *Ann Rheum Dis.* 1972;31:1-8.

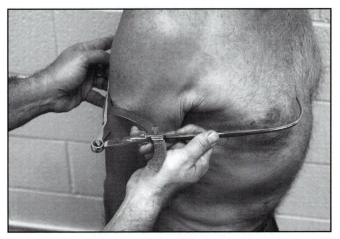

FIGURE 2-21. THORACIC DEPTH.

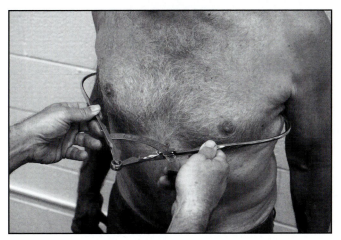

FIGURE 2-22. THORACIC WIDTH.

PULMONARY
SYSTEM

PULMONARY
SYSTEM

THORACIC EXCURSION MEASUREMENT
VIA CIRCUMFERENCE

TEST POSITION
- Standing

ACTION
- Place centimeter tape measure against skin, around chest, parallel to floor (so ends cross)
- Measure upper chest at 5th thoracic spinous process, 3rd intercostal (IC) space midclavicular line[1]
- Measure lower chest at 10th thoracic spinous process, xiphoid tip[1]
- Client takes full inspiration, then holds inhalation while examiner assesses circumference
- Client exhales fully and holds, while examiner assesses circumference
- Repeat inspiration and expiration 3 times and average
- Calculate thoracic excursion
- Thoracic excursion = end forced inspiration (cm) – end forced expiration (cm)

NORMAL FINDINGS
- Healthy adult males mean and standard deviation are as follows:
  - ✧ Upper: 3.6 cm (±0.6)[1]; Lower: 4.9 cm (±0.6)[1]

POSITIVE FINDINGS
- <1.7 cm: The low end of normal range[1]

SPECIAL CONSIDERATIONS
- Limited data on this technique, intraclass correlation coefficient = 0.86 (upper); 0.81 (lower)[1]
- Thoracic excursion is significantly correlated ($r = 0.71$) with vital capacity in adults with ankylosing spondylitis[2]
- Chest expansion significantly greater in exercisers (3.4 cm) vs nonexercisers (2.83 cm) with ankylosing spondylitis[2]
- In general chest expansion is greater in males vs females at all ages.[3]

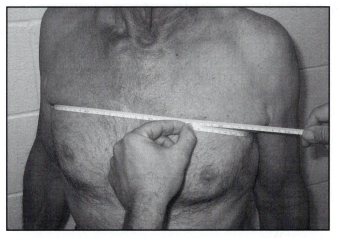

FIGURE 2-23. MEASUREMENT AT T5.

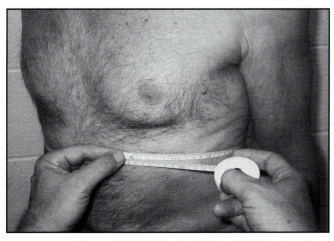

FIGURE 2-24. MEASUREMENT AT T10.

REFERENCES

1. Bockenhauer SE, Chen H, Julliard KN, Weedon J. Measuring thoracic excursion: reliability of the cloth measure technique. *J Am Osteopath Assoc.* 2007;107:191-196.

2. Fisher LR, Cawley MI, Holgate ST. Relation between chest expansion, pulmonary function, and exercise tolerance in patients with ankylosing spondylitis. *Ann Rheu Dis.* 1990;49:921-925.

3. Moll JM, Wright H. An objective clinical study of chest wall expansion. *Ann Rheum Dis.* 1972;31:1-8.

PULMONARY
SYSTEM

PALPATION OF TACTILE FREMITUS

TEST POSITION
- Seated

ACTION
- Place metacarpophalangeal joints (or ulnar hand surface) over posterior thorax between spinous processes and scapula
- Patient repeats "99" and examiner notes bilateral differences
- Repeat procedure: a) on anterior chest at supraclavicular area, b) lateral to sternum, c) below T4[1]

NORMAL FINDINGS
- Moderate vibration normally palpable unless assessing thick chest wall
- Usually stronger in upper chest between scapulae and spinous processes, and on right vs left[2]
- Low-pitched voice generates more fremitus than high-pitched voice[1]
- A thin chest wall allows for greater feel of fremitus than muscular or obese chest wall[1]

POSITIVE FINDINGS
- Increased or decreased fremitus during contralateral comparison warrants further investigation

SPECIAL CONSIDERATIONS
- Fremitus is palpable vibration of chest wall transmitted from the phonating larynx[3]
- Some examiners prefer unilateral palpation rather than simultaneous bilateral palpation
- Note fremitus as increased or reduced to a specific location[4]
- Abnormal fremitus should prompt auscultation of breath sounds, voice sounds
- Excellent interobserver agreement on fremitus (kappa = 0.86; 95% CI 0.74-0.97) and sensitivity and specificity is 0.76; (95% CI 0.63-0.87) and 0.88 (0.83-0.92), respectively, in those with pleural effusion[5]
- Other investigations have found much lower kappa values[6]

REFERENCES

1. Jarvis C. *Physical Examination and Health Assessment.* 5th ed. St. Louis, MO: Saunders-Elsevier; 2008

2. Finesilver C. Pulmonary assessment: what you need to know. *Prog Cardiovasc Nurs.* 2003;18:83-92.

3. Wilms JL, Schneiderman H, Algranati PS. *Physical Diagnosis: Bedside Evaluation of Diagnosis and Function.* Baltimore, MD: Williams & Wilkins; 1994.

4. Bickley LS, Szilagyi PG. *Bates' Guide to Physical Examination and History Taking.* 9th ed. Philadelphia, PA: Lippincott Williams & Wilkins; 2007.

5. Kalantri S, Joshi R, Lokhande T, et al. Accuracy and reliability of physical signs in the diagnosis of pleural effusion. *Respiratory Med.* 2007;101:431-438.

6. Maitre B, Similowski T, Derenne JP. Physical examination of the adult patient with respiratory disease: inspection and palpation. *Eur Respir J.* 1995; 8:1584-1593.

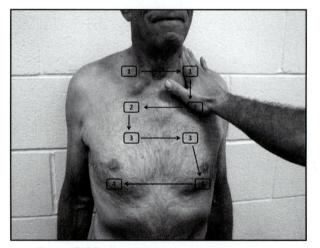

FIGURE 2-25. ASSESSMENT OF ANTERIOR FREMITUS.

PULMONARY SYSTEM

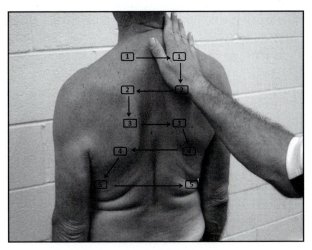

FIGURE 2-26. ASSESSMENT OF POSTERIOR FREMITUS.

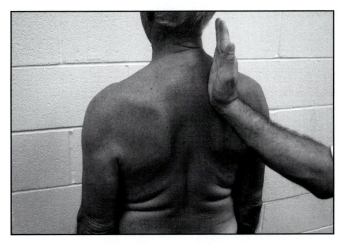

FIGURE 2-27. ASSESSMENT OF POSTERIOR FREMITUS.

PULMONARY
SYSTEM

PERCUSSION

TEST POSITION

- Posterior thorax percussion: seated; arms across chest
- Anterior thorax percussion: supine

ACTION

- Place nondominant distal interphalangeal joint of third finger in rib interspace and strike briskly and sharply with tip of dominant distal phalange, not allowing any other portion of hand to contact thorax[1]
- Strike each percussive note twice in the same location[1]
- Compare audible sounds to contralateral sides
- Percuss in one location, move across midline, and percuss at same level
- Move down, percuss, and cross midline again
- Posteriorly: Exclude percussion over scapulae
- Anteriorly: Percuss along midclavicular line; ask female clients to carefully move breast as necessary so right middle lobe may be assessed

NORMAL FINDINGS

- Sounds specific to anatomical locations should be heard only in those locations. If heard elsewhere, consider them abnormal[2]
- Anterior: Dullness noted in right midclavicular line from below T4 (nipple) inferiorly (over liver)
- Anterior: Dullness in 3rd to 5th left intercostal space (heart)

POSITIVE FINDINGS[2]

See Table 2-6 on the following page.

SPECIAL CONSIDERATIONS

- Vibrations are only transmitted from depths of 5 to 7 cm[2]
- If louder notes are needed, press harder, do not strike harder[1]

REFERENCES

1. Bickley LS, Szilagyi PG. *Bates' Guide to Physical Examination and History Taking.* 9th ed. Philadelphia, PA: Lippincott Williams & Wilkins; 2007.
2. Finesilver C. Pulmonary assessment: what you need to know. *Prog Cardiovasc Nurs.* 2003;18:83-92.

Table 2-6

A DESCRIPTION OF PERCUSSION SOUNDS

Type	Location	Intensity	Pitch	Quality	Duration	Sounds Like	Possible Pathologies
Resonant	Normal lung tissue	Loud	Low	Hollow	Long	Normal peripheral lung	
Hyper-resonant		Very loud[1]	Lowest		Longer[2]	Knocking on empty barrel[2]	Air trapping (asthma, emphysema, pneumothorax, pleural effusion)
Tympanic	Stomach or GI tract, air bubble[1]	Loud[1] Very loud[2]	Musical or high		Medium	Drum like	Large pneumothorax or emphysematous bleb
Dull	Liver[1]	Medium[1]	Medium-high	Thud like	Medium	Knocking on full barrel	Solid or fluid in air space due to pleural effusion, hemothorax, emphysema, consolidation, or mass[1,2]
Flat	Thigh[1]	Soft	High		Short	Duller than dull	Massive atelectasis, large pleural effusion, pneumonectomy[1,2]

Adapted from Bickley LS, Szilagyi PG. *Bates' Guide to Physical Examination and History Taking.* 9th ed. Philadelphia, PA: Lippincott Williams & Wilkins; 2007 and Finesilver C. Pulmonary assessment: what you need to know. *Prog Cardiovasc Nurs.* 2003;18:83-92.

PULMONARY SYSTEM

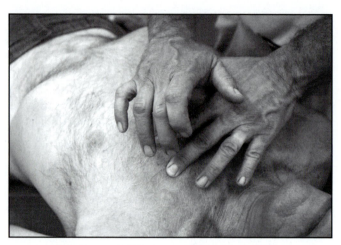

FIGURE 2-28. ANTERIOR PERCUSSION.

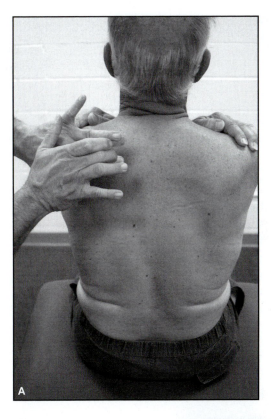

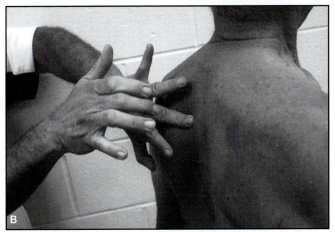

FIGURE 2-29. POSTERIOR PERCUSSION.

PULMONARY
SYSTEM

DIAPHRAGMATIC EXCURSION

TEST POSITION

- Seated with arms crossed anteriorly

ACTION

- Exhale, "hold it" while diaphragm rises
- Percuss posterior thorax in vertical line, medial to scapula[1]
- Mark where dullness replaces resonance on one side[1] to assess superior border
- Normal breathing, then "deep breath in and hold it[1]"
- Percuss posterior thorax in vertical line, medial and inferior to scapula[1] until resonance is replaced by dullness to assess inferior border of diaphragm
- Mark inferior border of diaphragm
- Mark extent of diaphragmatic excursion[2] and repeat for other side
- Anterior percussion occurs inferiorly from midclavicle moving laterally ~T4,5 bilaterally

NORMAL FINDINGS

- ~3 to 8 cm posterior diaphragmatic excursion in adults[1,2]
- Dullness heard anteriorly over heart and liver[1,2]

POSITIVE FINDINGS

- Smaller values, or unequal right vs left values[2]

SPECIAL CONSIDERATION

- Diaphragm may rise higher on right due to underlying liver[1]

REFERENCES

1. Jarvis C. *Physical Examination and Health Assessment*. 5th ed. St. Louis, MO: Saunders-Elsevier; 2008.
2. Bickley LS, Szilagyi PG. *Bates' Guide to Physical Examination and History Taking*. 9th ed. Philadelphia, PA: Lippincott Williams & Wilkins; 2007.

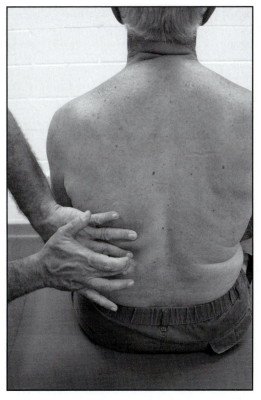

FIGURE 2-30. SUPERIOR BORDER.

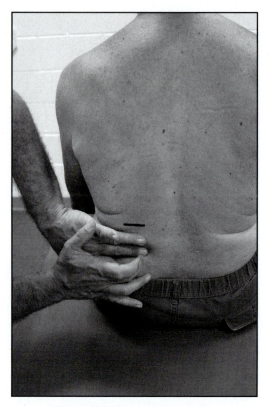

FIGURE 2-31. INFERIOR BORDER.

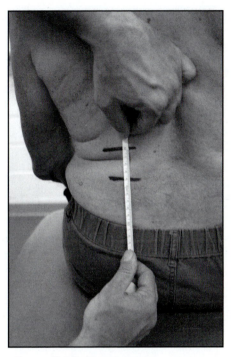

FIGURE 2-32. DIAPHRAGMATIC EXCURSION.

PULMONARY
SYSTEM

AUSCULTATION TECHNIQUE AND
NORMAL SOUNDS

TEST POSITION

- Seated; anterior and posterior thorax exposed as needed

ACTION

- Client performs deep breathing by mouth only when stethoscope head is placed against the skin; compare audible sounds to contralateral sides
- Posteriorly
  - ✧ Place stethoscope diaphragm in rib interspace beginning on left side of C7
  - ✧ Auscultate in one location, move across midline, and auscultate at same level for ≥1 full breath per location[1]
  - ✧ Move down, auscultate, and cross midline again; remain medial to scapular border

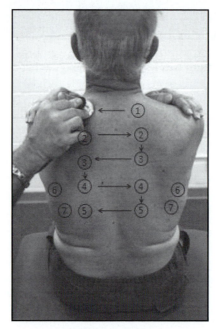

FIGURE 2-33. AUSCULTATION OF
POSTERIOR THORAX.

- If abnormal (adventitious) sounds are detected, "inch" stethoscope around area to clarify extent of involvement
- Difficult-to-hear sounds may be assessed by having patient take deeper breaths
- Anteriorly: Repeat pattern as above along midclavicular line; ask female clients to carefully move breast as necessary so right middle lobe may be assessed

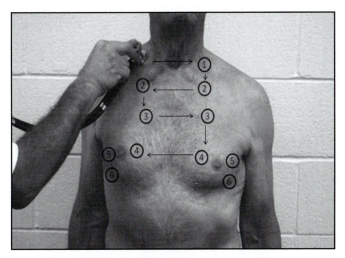

FIGURE 2-34. AUSCULTATION OF ANTERIOR THORAX.

NORMAL FINDINGS

- Appropriate intensity, pitch, quality, duration-based and side-to-side comparison[1]
- Crackles may be normally heard at lung bases in elderly and clear with position change or activity
- Refer to Table 2-7 on page 81 for normal breath sounds based on various locations in the thorax

PULMONARY
SYSTEM

POSITIVE FINDINGS

- Crackles (rales) defined by amplitude-intensity, pitch, duration[1] (Tables 2-8 and 2-9)
- Wheezes are defined by pitch, timing, and location[1] (Table 2-10)

SPECIAL CONSIDERATIONS

- Stethoscope diaphragm warmed with examiner hand
- Prevent hyperventilation by having client breathe only when stethoscope head is against skin, or with periodic breaks
- Always auscultate over skin, not over clothing
- Wet chest hair,[2] if necessary, to improve auscultation
- Crackles first appear at lung bases and spread upward as condition worsens
- Crackles noted in dependent areas predominate in expiration, although may be heard during inspiration
- Wheezes: Musical with many notes or a single note—musical snoring[2]
- Stridor is heard as an inspiratory crowing sound[2]
- Adventitious sounds may be heard at www.cvmbs.colostate.edu/clinsci/callan/breath_sounds.htm

REFERENCES

1. Bickley LS, Szilagyi PG. *Bates' Guide to Physical Examination and History Taking.* 9th ed. Philadelphia, PA: Lippincott Williams & Wilkins; 2007.
2. Jarvis C. *Physical Examination and Health Assessment.* 5th ed. St. Louis, MO: Saunders-Elsevier; 2008.

Table 2-7

NORMAL BREATH SOUNDS

Normal Sounds	Normally Heard Location	Caused by	Intensity	Pitch	Quality	Duration	Sounds Like
Tracheal	Trachea,[2] larynx[1]		Very loud[1,2]	High[1,2]	Harsh or hollow[2]	Equal inspiratory and expiratory[1,2]	
Bronchial (described as tracheal, tracheo-bronchial, tubular)	Mainstem bronchi	Turbulent airflow	Loud	High[1]	Harsh or hollow[2]	Longer expiratory vs inspiratory phase[1]	Tubular—air rushing through tube
Broncho-vesicular	Over mainstem bronchi, 1st and 2nd ICS,[1] and between scapulae[2]	Greater filtering of sounds by lung tissue	Moderate[2]	Moderate[1,2]	Less harsh	Equal inspiratory and expiratory phases[1]	
Vesicular	Peripheral lung fields anteriorly and posteriorly	Decreased turbulence	Soft[1]	Low[1,2]	Rustling[2]	Longer inspiratory phase, short expiratory phase[1]	Wind rushing through trees[2]

Adapted from Bickley LS, Szilagyi PG. Szilagyi PG. *Bates' Guide to Physical Examination and History Taking.* 9th ed. Philadelphia, PA: Lippincott Williams & Wilkins; 2007 and Jarvis C. *Physical Examination and Health Assessment.* 5th ed. St. Louis, MO: Saunders-Elsevier; 2008.

Table 2-8

DESCRIPTION OF CRACKLES

Type	Duration	Amplitude	Intensity	Pitch
Fine crackles	Discontinuous, brief	Low	Soft	High
Course crackles	Discontinuous, longer	High	Louder	Low

Table 2-9

CHARACTERISTICS OF CRACKLES

For crackles, note number, timing in breathing cycle, location, and persistence from breath to breath, changes after coughing, or position change.[1]

	Late Inspiratory Crackles	Early Inspiratory Crackles	Midinspiratory and Expiratory Crackles
Number	Profuse	Few	Profuse
Timing	Mid → Late inspiration	Early inspiration	Midinspiration and expiration
Location	Bases → Upward		
Persistence	From breath to breath		
Seen in:	Interstitial lung disease, fibrosis, CHF	Chronic bronchitis, asthma	Bronchiectasis

Adapted from Bickley LS, Szilagyi PG. *Bates' Guide to Physical Examination and History Taking.* 9th ed. Philadelphia, PA: Lippincott Williams & Wilkins; 2007

Table 2-10

DESCRIPTION OF WHEEZES

For wheezes (rhonchi), note when and where they are heard, as well as if and how they change with coughing or deep breathing.[1]

	Pitch	Timing	Location	Changes With Coughing or Deep Breathing	Suggests
Wheezes	High[2]	Inspiration and expiration or expiration only[2]	Various	May clear with coughing[2]	Very narrowed airways due to bronchospasm, edema, foreign body[1]
Rhonchi	Low[2]	Inspiration and expiration (more prominent)	Heard best over large airways	Secretions in large airways[1] May clear with coughing[1]	Single to diffuse airway obstruction
Stridor	High	Inspiration	Louder in neck[2]	Obstructed airway	Medical emergency

Adapted from Bickley LS, Szilagyi PG. *Bates' Guide to Physical Examination and History Taking.* 9th ed. Philadelphia, PA: Lippincott Williams & Wilkins; 2007 and Jarvis C. *Physical Examination and Health Assessment.* 5th ed. St. Louis, MO: Saunders-Elsevier; 2008.

AUSCULTATION OF TRANSMITTED VOICE SOUNDS

TEST POSITION
- Posterior thorax: seated
- Anterior thorax: supine

ACTION
- Abnormally located bronchovesicular or bronchial sounds can be further examined by assessing transmitted sounds[1]
- Say "99" or "Ee" or whisper "1, 2, 3" when the stethoscope diaphragm is placed upon the thorax
- Auscultation pattern is as described on pages 78 and 79

Table 2-11

NORMAL AND POSITIVE FINDINGS

Patient	Test	Normal Finding	Positive Finding	Suggestive of
Says 99, 99, 99	Bronchophony	Indistinguishable sounds/ muffled	"99" clearly heard	Increased lung density[2]
Says Ee, Ee, Ee	Egophony	Muffled long-E sound	Hard "Aaaa" sound	Consolidation[1]
Whispers 1, 2, 3	Whispering pectoriloquy	Faint or indistinct	1, 2, 3 clearly heard	Consolidation[2]

Adapted from Bickley LS, Szilagyi PG. *Bates' Guide to Physical Examination and History Taking.* 9th ed. Philadelphia, PA: Lippincott Williams & Wilkins; 2007 and Jarvis C. *Physical Examination and Health Assessment.* 5th ed. St. Louis, MO: Saunders-Elsevier; 2008.

SPECIAL CONSIDERATIONS
- Consolidation is noted via increased tactile and vocal fremitus[3]
- Consolidation prevents voice sounds from spreading out through lung tissue, resulting in intensified sound transmission[2]
- These tests have been shown to have low kappa values and low sensitivity in clients with pneumonia[4]

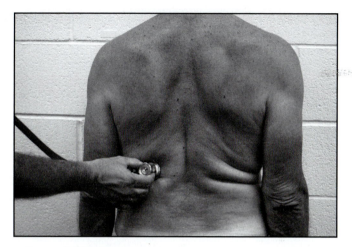

FIGURE 2-35. AUSCULTATION OF TRANSMITTED VOICE SOUNDS.

REFERENCES

1. Bickley LS, Szilagyi PG. *Bates' Guide to Physical Examination and History Taking.* 9th ed. Philadelphia, PA: Lippincott Williams & Wilkins; 2007.
2. Jarvis C. *Physical Examination and Health Assessment.* 5th ed. St. Louis, MO: Saunders-Elsevier; 2008.
3. Finesilver C. Pulmonary assessment: what you need to know. *Prog Cardiovasc Nurs.* 2003;18:83-92.
4. Wipf JE, Lipsky BA, Hirschmann JV, et al. Diagnosing pneumonia by physical examination. *Arch Inter Med.* 1999;159:1082-1087.

PULMONARY
SYSTEM

OXYGEN SATURATION

TEST POSITION
- Seated or supine
- Clean finger and fingernail

ACTION
- Place probe on client's index finger

NORMAL FINDINGS

Table 2-12

SpO₂ VALUES

Population	SpO_2 Value	Activity
Healthy adults	≥95%	Rest, sleep, exertion
Adults with COPD[1,2]	90%	Rest, sleep, exertion, pulmonary rehabilitation
Infants/children beyond age of oxygen-induced retinopathy[3]	≥95%	Rest, sleep, exertion

POSITIVE FINDINGS
- SpO_2 values lower than normal

SPECIAL CONSIDERATION
- Check pulse oximeter product literature regarding accuracy during physical activity

REFERENCES

1. American Thoracic Society/European Respiratory Society Task Force. Standards for the diagnosis and management of patients with COPD [Internet]. Version 1.2. New York: American Thoracic Society; 2004 [updated 2005 September 8]. http://www.thoracic.org/clinical/copd-guide-lines/resources/copddoc.pdf. Accessed July 23, 2010.
2. ATS statement: guidelines for the six-minute walk test. *Am J Respir Crit Care Med.* 2002;166:111-117. http://www.thoracic.org/statements/resources/pfet/sixminute.pdf. Accessed July 23, 2010.

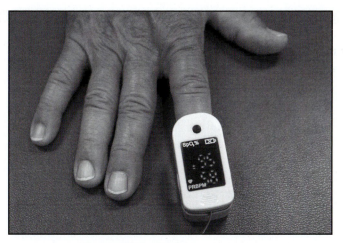

FIGURE 2-36. OXYGEN SATURATION.

3. ATS statement: statement on the care of the child with chronic lung disease of infancy and childhood. *Am J Respir Crit Care Med.* 2003;168:356-396. http://www.atsjournals.org/cgi/reprint/168/3/356? maxtoshow=&HITS=10&hits=10&RESULTFORMAT=&searchd=1&FIRSTINDEX=0&volume=168&firstpage=356&resourcetype=HWCIT. Accessed April 14, 2009.

CHEST DISORDERS

TEST POSITION
- Seated

SPECIAL CONSIDERATION
See Table 2-13 on the following pages.

Table 2-13

FINDINGS DURING AN EVALUATION OF THE RESPIRATORY SYSTEM

Condition	Tracheal Position	Tactile Fremitus Over Involved Area Transmitted Voice Sounds	Percussion Over Involved Area	Breath Sounds Over Involved Area	Adventitious Sounds Over Involved Area
Normal	Normal[1]	Normal, equal bilaterally[2]	Resonant[2]	Normal tracheal, bronchial, bronchovesicular, and vesicular sounds	None[2] Inspiratory crackles at bases may be considered normal in elderly[1]
Asthma	Normal[1]	Decreased[2]	Resonant Hyperresonant if chronic[2]	Wheezes make breath sounds unclear[1]	Wheezes,[2] perhaps crackles
Atelectasis	May shift toward involved side[1,2]	Usually absent over atelectatic area[1,2] Transmitted sounds may be heard over right apex in right upper lobe atelectasis[1]	Dull[2]	Usually absent, decreased[2]; tracheal sounds may be transmitted sounds to right apex	None[1]

(continued)

Table 2-13 (continued)

FINDINGS DURING AN EVALUATION OF THE RESPIRATORY SYSTEM

Condition	Tracheal Position	Tactile Fremitus Over Involved Area Transmitted Voice Sounds	Percussion Over Involved Area	Breath Sounds Over Involved Area	Adventitious Sounds Over Involved Area
Pneumo-thorax	May shift away from involved side[1,2]	Decreased to absent[2]	Hyperresonant[2] to tympanic[1]	Decreased or absent[2]	None[2] or possible pleural friction rub
Pleural effusion	May shift away from involved side[1,2]	Absent or decreased[2] Perhaps increased toward top of large effusion	Flat or dull[2]	Absent or decreased[2] Perhaps heard toward top of large effusion	None[2] or possible pleural friction rub[1]
Consolid-ation	Normal[1]	Increased[1] with posi-tive transmitted voice sound tests	Dull[1]	Bronchial[1]	Late inspiratory crackles

(continued)

Table 2-13 (continued)

FINDINGS DURING AN EVALUATION OF THE RESPIRATORY SYSTEM

Condition	Tracheal Position	Tactile Fremitus Over Involved Area Transmitted Voice Sounds	Percussion Over Involved Area	Breath Sounds Over Involved Area	Adventitious Sounds Over Involved Area
Left-sided heart failure	Normal[1]	Normal[2]	Resonant[2]	Vesicular[2]	Late inspiratory crackles[2] Wheezes possible
Bronchitis	Normal[1]	Normal[2]	Resonant[2]	Vesicular[2]	None[2] → Early inspiratory, perhaps expiratory coarse crackles[1] Wheezes and rhonchi are possible[1]
Emphysema	Normal[1]	Decreased[2]	Hyperresonant[2] and diffuse[1]	Absent or decreased[2]	None[2] and/or bronchitic symptoms[1]

Adapted from Bickley LS, Szilagyi PG. *Bates' Guide to Physical Examination and History Taking.* 9th ed. Philadelphia, PA: Lippincott Williams & Wilkins; 2007 and Jarvis C. *Physical Examination and Health Assessment.* 5th ed. St. Louis, MO: Saunders-Elsevier; 2008.

PULMONARY SYSTEM

DYSPNEA WITH ACTIVITIES OF DAILY LIVING

TEST POSITION

- Walking or daily tasks

ACTION

- Show Modified MRC Dyspnea Scale and ask for dyspnea rating
- Rating of 1 to 5 prompts questioning related to dyspnea

NORMAL FINDING

- None

POSITIVE FINDINGS

- "1 to 5" rating

Table 2-14

MODIFIED MRC DYSPNEA SCALE[1]

Grade	Degree	Characteristics
1	Slight	Shortness of breath when hurrying on level ground or climbing a slight incline
2	Moderate	Walks slower than others of the same age on level ground because of breathlessness
3	Moderately severe	Stops because of breathlessness when walking at one pace on level ground
4	Severe	Stops for breath after 100 yards or after a few minutes walking on level ground
5	Very severe	Housebound or breathless when dressing or undressing

Reprinted with permission from Darbee JC, Ohtake PJ. Outcome measures in cardiopulmonary physical therapy: medical research council (MRC) dyspnea scale. *Cardiopulm Phys Ther J.* 2006;17:29-36.

Table 2-15

KEY QUESTIONS IN EVALUATION OF DYSPNEA[2]

Question	Possible Pathophysiology
Associated only with exertion?	Heart failure, restrictive or obstructive lung disease
Associated with exertion and occurs at night? Cough and wheeze?	Asthma or heart failure
Associated with exertion, chest, and/or neck discomfort and concurrent nausea or diaphoresis?	Angina pectoris
Worse when assuming upright position?	Liver disease with arterio-venous shunts at the lung bases (platypnea)
Present in the lateral decubitus position?	Unilateral lung or pleural disease (trepopnea)
Fast onset when supine, relieved by lateral or upright positioning?	Bilateral phrenic nerve dysfunction

Reprinted with permission from Hudson LD, Murray JF, Petty TL, et al. Frontline assessment of common pulmonary presentations. The Snowdrift Pulmonary Foundation, 2001.

PULMONARY SYSTEM

SPECIAL CONSIDERATION

- MRC scale has very good interrater reliability (Kw = 0.92) and acceptable concurrent validity (r = 0.53-0.87)[1]

REFERENCES

1. Darbee JC, Ohtake PJ. Outcome measures in cardiopulmonary physical therapy: medical research council (MRC) dyspnea scale. *Cardiopulm Phys Ther J*. 2006;17:29-36.
2. Hudson LD, Murray JF, Petty TL, et al. Frontline assessment of common pulmonary presentations. The Snowdrift Pulmonary Foundation, 2001.

PULMONARY SYSTEM

DYSPNEA AT REST

TEST POSITION

- Seated, resting

ACTION

- Show rating scale and ask for current rating[1]
- Select a number from 0 to 10 that represents your current feeling of shortness of breath

  | 0 | 1 | 2 | 3 | 4 | 5 | 6 | 7 | 8 | 9 | 10 |

NORMAL FINDINGS

- "0" = nothing at all[2]

POSITIVE FINDINGS

- 0.5 = very, very slight; 3 = moderate; 5 = severe; 7 = very severe; 9 = very, very severe; 10 = maximal[2]

SPECIAL CONSIDERATIONS

- Changes in modified 0-10 Borg Scale correlated highly with changes in pulmonary function tests[2]
- Dyspnea is "a subjective experience of breathing discomfort that consists of qualitatively distinct sensations that vary in intensity"[2]
- Chronic dyspnea is dyspnea that lasts longer than 1 month[2]
- Test-retest correlation ($r = 0.93$)[1]
- Low correlations between FEV_1, O_2 saturation, and dyspnea at rest[1]
- Present dyspnea and usual dyspnea scores do not correlate[1]
- Visual Analog Scales with a 10-cm length can be used

REFERENCES

1. Gift AG, Narsavage G. Validity of the numeric rating scale as a measure of dyspnea. *Am J Crit Care.* 1998;7:200-204.
2. Kendrick KR, Baxi SC, Smith RM. Usefulness of the modified 0-10 Scale in assessing the degree of dyspnea in patients with COPD and asthma. *J Emerg Nurs.* 2000;26:216-222.
3. American Thoracic Society. Dyspnea. Mechanisms, assessment, and management: a consensus statement. *Am J Respir Crit Care Med.* 1999;159:321-340.

DYSPNEA DURING ACTIVITY

TEST POSITION
- Treadmill or cycle ergometer

ACTION
- Show rating scale[1]
- Select a number from 0 to 10 that represents your current feeling of shortness of breath

  0   1   2   3   4   5   6   7   8   9   10

NORMAL FINDINGS
- Dyspnea may increase with increasing intensities

POSITIVE FINDINGS
- Ratings causing patient to stop exercise[2]
- Healthy individuals and those with air flow limitations provide similar ratings when terminating exercise tests; however, those with air flow limitations stop at significantly lower workload intensities[3]

SPECIAL CONSIDERATIONS
- Verbal dyspnea scale correlated highly with respiratory rate ($r = 0.95$), heart rate ($r = 0.90$), and SBP ($r = 0.95$)[2]
- Dyspnea scales should be used during ADL, during each minute of exercise testing so discrete changes may be noted[4]
- The numeric rating scale and the visual analog scale are highly correlated measures of dyspnea[1]

REFERENCES
1. Gift AG, Narsavage G. Validity of the numeric rating scale as a measure of dyspnea. *Am J Crit Care.* 1998;7:200-204.
2. Saracino A, Weiland T, Dent A, Jolly B. Validation of a verbal rating scale for breathlessness amongst patients referred for cardiac stress tests. *Heart Lung Circ.* 2008;17:305-312.
3. Killian KJ, Leblanc P, Martin DH, Summers E, Jones NL, Campbell EJ. Exercise capacity and ventilatory, circulatory, and symptom limitation in patients with chronic airflow limitation. *Am Rev Respir Dis.* 1992;146:935-940.
4. Mahler DA. Mechanisms and measurement of dyspnea in chronic obstructive pulmonary disease. *Proc Am Thorac Soc.* 2006;3:234-238.

PULMONARY SYSTEM

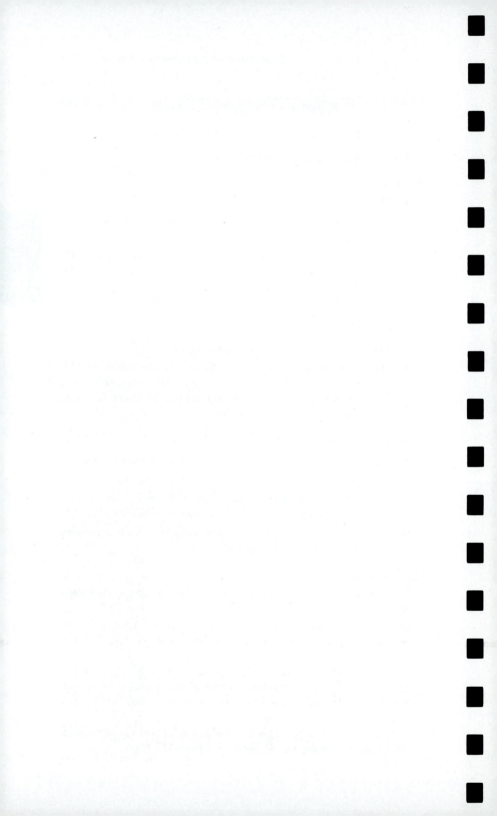

Examination of the Abdomen

ABDOMEN

INSPECTION

TEST POSITION

- Supine on exam table, head on pillow, arms at sides, knees bent to 90° or supported by pillows (for relaxation) with examiner standing at right side

ACTION

- Inspect for contour, symmetry, umbilicus, skin integrity, and pulsation or movement

NORMAL FINDINGS

- Contour: Flat or rounded
- Symmetry: Bilaterally
- Umbilicus: Midline, inverted
- Skin: Smooth, similar color overall
- Pulsation or movement: Pulsation from the aorta, peristalsis, respiration; should rise and fall rhythmically with respirations

POSITIVE FINDINGS

- Contour: Protuberance or distension of the abdomen may indicate ascites or obesity; sunken may indicate emaciation.
- Symmetry: Localized bulging, masses, hernias
- Umbilicus: Protruding, discolored, or inflamed
- Skin: Redness, jaundice, tautness, striae, rashes, angiomas, scars, poor turgor, dilated veins
- Bulging along the inguinal canal when the patient is asked to cough suggests an inguinal hernia.
- Pulsation or movement: Marked pulsation of aorta, distended abdomen with marked peristalsis
- Cullen's sign: Ecchymosis around the umbilicus due to retroperitoneal hemorrhage
- Grey Turner's sign: Ecchymosis around the flanks due to retroperitoneal hemorrhage

SPECIAL CONSIDERATIONS

- Use warm room, warm stethoscope, and warm hands

O'Connell DG, O'Connell JK, Hinman MR.
Special Tests of the Cardiopulmonary, Vascular and Gastrointestinal Systems (pp 98-128).
© 2011 SLACK Incorporated

- Consider the normal anatomy as presented in Table 3-1
- Description of abdominal pain in Table 3-2

Table 3-1

ORGAN LOCATION IN THE ABDOMEN

Right Upper Quadrant (RUQ)	*Left Upper Quadrant (LUQ)*
Liver	Stomach
Gallbladder	Spleen
Right kidney	Left lobe of liver
Head of pancreas	Left kidney
Parts of colon	Body of pancreas
	Parts of colon
Possible Cause of Pain: *Acute cholecystitis, biliary colic, acute hepatitis, duodenal ulcer, right lower lobe pneumonia*	**Possible Cause of Pain:** *Gastritis, acute pancreatitis, splenic pathology, left lower lobe pneumonia*
Right Lower Quadrant (RLQ)	*Left Lower Quadrant (LLQ)*
Appendix	Sigmoid and descending colon
Right ureter	Left ureter
Cecum	Spermatic cord
Spermatic cord	
Possible Cause of Pain: *Appendicitis, cecal diverticulitis, ectopic pregnancy, tubo-ovarian abscess, ruptured ovarian cyst, ovarian torsion*	**Possible Cause of Pain:** *Diverticulitis, ectopic pregnancy, tubo-ovarian abscess, ruptured ovarian cyst, ovarian torsion*

Midline

Aorta

Bladder (if distended)

Uterus (if enlarged)

Possible Cause of Pain: *Appendicitis (early), gastroenteritis, myocardial ischemia or infarction, pancreatitis*

Adapted from Jarvis C. *Physical Examination and Health Assessment.* 5th ed. St. Louis, MO: Saunders-Elsevier; 2008; Walker HK, Hall WD, Hurst JW, eds. *Clinical Methods: The History, Physical, and Laboratory Examinations.* 3rd ed. London: Butterworths; 1990; and White MJ, Counselman FL. Troubleshooting acute abdominal pain. Part 1. *Emerg Med.* 2002:20;34-42.

Table 3-2

DESCRIPTION OF ABDOMINAL PAIN

- Visceral pain
  - ✧ Hollow abdominal organs (intestine, biliary tree contract forcefully or are distended)
  - ✧ Solid organs (liver) pain when capsule is stretched
  - ✧ Difficult to localize
  - ✧ Often near midline at appropriate level
  - ✧ Gnawing, burning, cramping, or aching
  - ✧ When severe—sweating, pallor, nausea, vomiting, restlessness
- Parietal pain
  - ✧ Originates in parietal peritoneum, caused by inflammation
  - ✧ Steady aching pain more severe than visceral pain is precisely located over structure
  - ✧ Worsens with movement or coughing
- Referred pain
  - ✧ Pain felt in more distant sites innervated at approximately the same spinal levels as disordered structure
  - ✧ Pain seems to travel from original location to distant location
  - ✧ Superficial or deep, but well localized
  - ✧ Referred to abdomen from chest, spine, or pelvis, or from abdomen to shoulder or back

Adapted from Jarvis C. *Physical Examination and Health Assessment.* 5th ed. St. Louis, MO: Saunders-Elsevier; 2008; Walker HK, Hall WD, Hurst JW, eds. *Clinical Methods: The History, Physical, and Laboratory Examinations.* 3rd ed. London: Butterworths; 1990; and White MJ, Counselman FL. Troubleshooting acute abdominal pain. Part 1. *Emerg Med.* 2002:20;34-42.

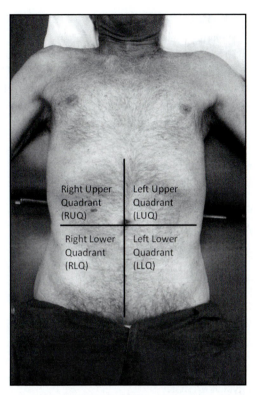

FIGURE 3-1. ANTERIOR QUADRANTS.

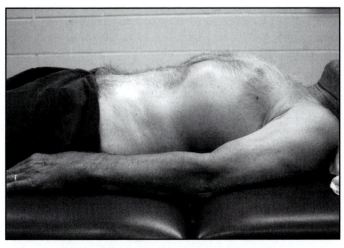

FIGURE 3-2. LATERAL ABDOMINAL CONTOUR.

AUSCULTATION OF THE ABDOMINAL VASCULATURE

TEST POSITION

- Supine on exam table, head on pillow, arms at sides, knees bent to 90° or supported by pillows (for relaxation) with examiner standing at right side

ACTION

- Hold stethoscope diaphragm firmly over the aorta, renal, iliac, splenic, and femoral arteries
- Begin in the URQ and work clockwise through all quadrants.[1]

NORMAL FINDINGS

- Bowel sounds are normal

POSITIVE FINDINGS

- Bruits, or loud blowing sounds found with systole or diastole are due to arterial atherosclerosis and represent turbulent blood flow[2]
- Bruits with systole may be normal but referral and additional testing is typical
- Renal bruits may be found in those with hypertension

SPECIAL CONSIDERATION

- Bruits are often associated with hypertension or aortic aneurysms

REFERENCES

1. Jarvis C. *Physical Examination and Health Assessment.* 5th ed. St. Louis, MO: Saunders-Elsevier; 2008.
2. Walker HK, Hall WD, Hurst JW, eds. *Clinical Methods: The History, Physical, and Laboratory Examinations.* 3rd ed. London: Butterworths; 1990.

ABDOMEN

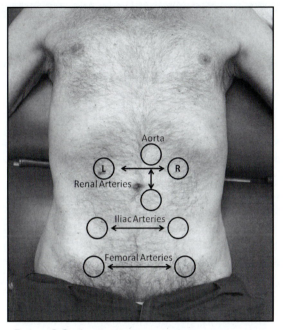

FIGURE 3-3. AUSCULTATION OF AORTIC, RENAL, ILIAC, AND FEMORAL ARTERIES.

ABDOMEN

PERCUSSION OF THE ABDOMEN

TEST POSITION
- Supine on exam table, head on pillow, arms at sides, knees bent to 90° or supported by pillows (for relaxation) with examiner standing at right side

ACTION
- Assess for the amount and distribution of gas in the abdomen, rule out ascites, and identify specific organs
- Begin in URQ, move clockwise to cover all quadrants[1]
- Technique[2]
  - ◇ Metacarpal interphalangeal joint of third finger of left hand pressed firmly on the abdomen; remainder of hand not touching the abdomen
  - ◇ Flexed distal interphalangeal joint (DIP) of the middle finger of the right hand strikes the DIP of the left perpendicularly, like a hammer
  - ◇ Use wrist action only, not the entire arm

NORMAL FINDINGS
- Tympany (hollow sounds) suggests gas in the gastrointestinal tract[3]
- Dullness represents fluids or solids[3]
- Flat or soft, high-pitched sounds generally heard over bones, muscles, and tumors
- Dullness (low amplitude, no resonance) heard over solid organs[3]
- Tympany (drum-like sound with resonance) over air-filled bowel or lung[3]

POSITIVE FINDINGS
- Ascites (intra-abdominal fluid): In supine, the belly may be rounded and the flanks bulging; there will be tympany in the central, ventral abdomen with dullness in the periphery; after 1 minute of side lying, tympany will be noted superiorly and dullness inferiorly.

SPECIAL CONSIDERATION
- Large, dull areas may be associated with pregnancy, ovarian tumor, or distended bladder[4]

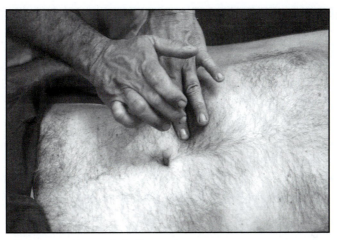

FIGURE 3-4. PERCUSSION OF ABDOMEN.

ABDOMEN

REFERENCES

1. Walker HK, Hall WD, Hurst JW, eds. *Clinical Methods: The History, Physical, and Laboratory Examinations.* 3rd ed. London: Butterworths; 1990.

2. Tryniszewski C, ed. *Mosby's Expert 10-Minute Physical Examinations.* 2nd ed. St. Louis, MO: Elsevier Health Sciences; 2004.

3. Urbano FL, Fedorowski JJ. Medical percussion. *Hospital Physician.* September 2000;31-36.   http://www.hpboardreview.com/pdf/hp_sep00_percus.pdf. Accessed on July 1, 2010.

4. Bickley LS, Szilagyi PG. *Bates' Guide to Physical Examination and History Taking.* 9th ed. Philadelphia, PA: Lippincott Williams & Wilkins; 2007.

LIGHT PALPATION OF THE ABDOMEN

TEST POSITION

- Supine on exam table, head on pillow, arms at sides, knees bent to 90° or supported by pillows (for relaxation) with examiner standing at right side

ACTION

- Place right hand fingertips flat on the abdomen and depress approximately 1 cm
- Circle fingers in a rotary motion, then move to the next area, repeating sequence in right and left upper and lower quadrants

NORMAL FINDINGS

- Voluntary guarding secondary to being ticklish, tense, or cold; crepitus of the abdominal wall suggesting gas or fluid in subcutaneous tissue

POSITIVE FINDINGS

- Involuntary rigidity resulting in a constant hardness of the muscles; tenderness may suggest peritoneal inflammation

SPECIAL CONSIDERATIONS

- Assess superficial musculature and determine an overall impression of the abdomen
- Examine last the area reported as tender

REFERENCES

1. Jarvis C. *Physical Examination and Health Assessment.* 5th ed. St. Louis, MO: Saunders-Elsevier; 2008.
2. Blank-Reid C. Abdominal trauma: dealing with the damage. *Nursing.* 2004;34(9):36-41.

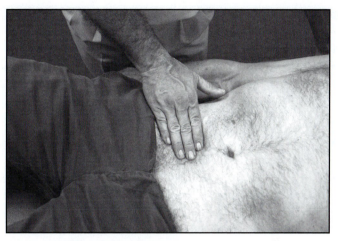

FIGURE 3-5. LIGHT ABDOMINAL PALPATION.

ABDOMEN

DEEP PALPATION OF THE ABDOMEN

TEST POSITION

- Supine on exam table, head on pillow, arms at sides, knees bent to 90° or supported by pillows (for relaxation) with examiner standing at right side

ACTION

- Assess for the size, location, consistency, and mobility of organs to determine masses or tenderness
- Place 4 fingers of the right hand flatly on the abdomen and depress 5 to 8 cm (2 to 3 inches)[1]
- Circle fingers in a rotary motion, then move to the next area, repeating through all 4 quadrants
- In obese patients, use a 2-hand technique by placing one hand on top of the other and pushing with the top hand, keeping the bottom hand relaxed to feel the organs.[1]

NORMAL FINDINGS

- No guarding, tenderness, masses, or enlargement of organs

POSITIVE FINDINGS

- Tenderness, masses, enlargement of organs, tissues, or muscles

SPECIAL CONSIDERATIONS

- Rebound tenderness produces more pain when fingers are lifted from the site
- Examine last the area reported as tender

REFERENCE

1. Jarvis C. *Physical Examination and Health Assessment.* 5th ed. St. Louis, MO: Saunders-Elsevier; 2008.

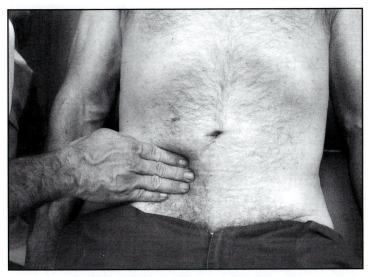

FIGURE 3-6. DEEP PALPATION USING ONE HAND.

ABDOMEN

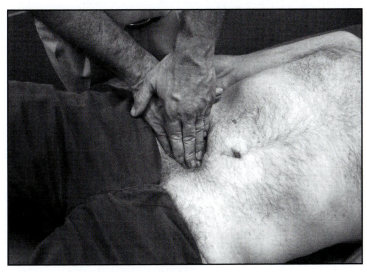

FIGURE 3-7. DEEP PALPATION USING 2 HANDS.

DEEP PALPATION OF THE ABDOMEN— BIMANUAL TECHNIQUE FOR THE LIVER

TEST POSITION

- Supine on exam table, head on pillow, arms at sides, knees bent to 90° or supported by pillows (for relaxation) with examiner standing at right side

ACTION

- Assess for the size, location, consistency, and mobility of the liver to determine masses or tenderness
- Place left hand under patient's back parallel to the lowest ribs
- Place fingers of the right hand in the RUQ, parallel to the midline
- Upon deep inhalation, push down firmly under the costal margin

NORMAL FINDINGS

- A smooth, firm edge of the liver may be felt by the right hand
- Not being able to palpate the liver is also normal

POSITIVE FINDINGS

- Edge of liver extending beyond 1 to 2 cm of the costal margin indicates enlargement
- Heart failure: Enlarged, soft, smooth, and tender.
- Metastasis: Enlarged, hard, irregular or nodular, nontender

SPECIAL CONSIDERATION

- The liver is located in the RUQ between ribs 7 and 11

REFERENCE

1. Jarvis C. *Physical Examination and Health Assessment.* 5th ed. St. Louis, MO: Saunders-Elsevier; 2008.

ABDOMEN

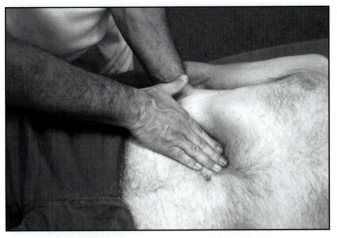

FIGURE 3-8. BIMANUAL TECHNIQUE.

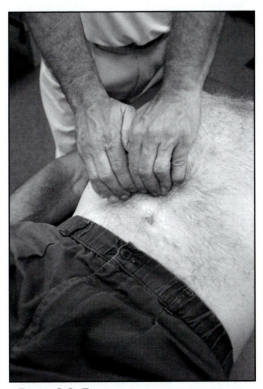

FIGURE 3-9. TWO-HAND OR HOOK TECHNIQUE.

DEEP PALPATION OF THE ABDOMEN— BIMANUAL TECHNIQUE FOR THE SPLEEN

TEST POSITION

- Supine on exam table, head on pillow, arms at sides, knees bent to 90° or supported by pillows (for relaxation) with examiner standing at right side

ACTION

- Assess for the size, location, consistency, and mobility of the spleen to determine masses or tenderness
- Reach across client and position left hand on the client's left side at the lowest ribs
- Place right hand's fingers inferior to costal margin, pointing toward axilla, and press firmly as the patient takes a deep breath

NORMAL FINDINGS

- Not palpable

POSITIVE FINDINGS

- Palpable and firm, extending below the costal margin.

SPECIAL CONSIDERATIONS

- The spleen is located in the LUQ between ribs 9 and 11[1]
- Specificity for splenomegaly during a routine examine = 98%; sensitivity = 27%[2]

REFERENCES

1. Jarvis C. *Physical Examination and Health Assessment.* 5th ed. St. Louis, MO: Saunders-Elsevier; 2008.
2. Grover SA, Barkun AN, Sackett DL. Does this patient have splenomegaly? *JAMA.* 1993;10:2218-2221.

ABDOMEN

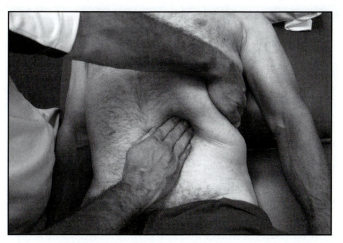

FIGURE 3-10. BIMANUAL SPLEEN PALPATION.

DEEP PALPATION OF THE ABDOMEN— BIMANUAL TECHNIQUE FOR THE KIDNEYS

TEST POSITION

- Supine on exam table, head on pillow, arms at sides, knees bent to 90° or supported by pillows (for relaxation) with examiner standing at right side

ACTION

- Assess for the size, location, consistency, and mobility of the kidneys to determine masses or tenderness
- Place one hand under the back and one hand on top of the abdomen just below the costal margin
- Press the 2 hands together firmly as the client inhales deeply

NORMAL FINDINGS

- Might be able to palpate the smooth, rounded, lower pole of the kidney

POSITIVE FINDINGS

- Enlarged kidney; may have nodules or tenderness

SPECIAL CONSIDERATION

- Left kidney is normally 1 cm higher than right[1]

REFERENCE

1. Jarvis C. *Physical Examination and Health Assessment.* 5th ed. St. Louis, MO: Saunders-Elsevier; 2008.

ABDOMEN

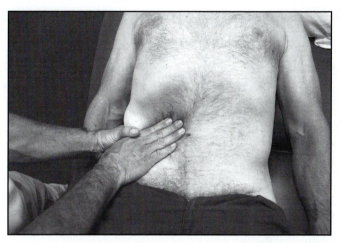

FIGURE 3-11. BIMANUAL KIDNEY PALPATION.

ABDOMEN

DEEP PALPATION OF THE AORTA

TEST POSITION

- Supine on exam table, head on pillow, arms at sides, knees bent to 90° or supported by pillows (for relaxation) with examiner standing at right side

ACTION

- Assess for the size, location, and pulsation of the aorta
- Place the palms of both hands on the patient's abdomen, with the index fingers pointing toward the head, just above the umbilicus and slightly left of midline
- Press down firmly to locate the pulsating aorta

NORMAL FINDINGS

- Aorta width ~2.5 cm (1 inch or ~2 fingertip widths)
- Pulsation should be felt anteriorly

POSITIVE FINDINGS

- Wide aortic pulsations (≥4 cm) or lateral pulsations may indicate abdominal aortic aneurysm (AAA) and should be referred
- Width, not pulsation intensity, is most important

SPECIAL CONSIDERATIONS

- Sensitivity of palpation = 68%; specificity = 75%[1]
- Sensitivity increases with the size of the AAA up to .82% for AAA >5 cm[1]
- Sensitivity in subjects with less than a 40-inch waistline = 91%[1]
- Positive predictive value from palpation of AAA >3 cm = 43%[2]

REFERENCES

1. Fink HA, Lederle FA, Roth CS, Bowles CA, Nelson DB, Haas MA. The accuracy of physical examination to detect abdominal aortic aneurysm. *Arch Intern Med.* 2000;160:833-836.
2. Lederle FA, Simel DL. The rational clinical examination: does this patient have abdominal aortic aneurysm? *JAMA.* 1999;281:77-82.

ABDOMEN

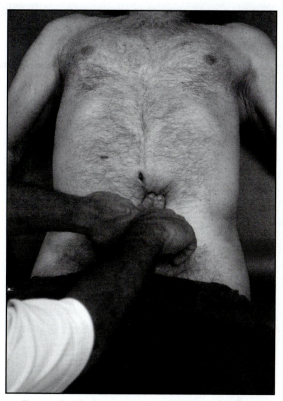

FIGURE 3-12. PALPATION OF AORTIC PULSATION.

ABDOMEN

BLUMBERG'S SIGN (REBOUND TENDERNESS)

TEST POSITION

- Supine on exam table, head on pillow, arms at sides, knees bent to 90° or supported by pillows (for relaxation) with examiner standing at right side

ACTION

- When assessing abdominal tenderness, place right hand perpendicular to the abdomen and push down slowly and deeply, then release quickly but smoothly[1]

NORMAL FINDINGS

- No pain with release of downward pressure

POSITIVE FINDINGS

- Pain and rigidity, facial grimace, or spasm upon release of pressure

SPECIAL CONSIDERATIONS

- Palpation of the LLQ may produce rebound tenderness in the RLQ in appendicitis
- Rovsing's sign: Pain when ascending colon is manually palpated
- Further testing, such as blood work and ultrasound, are necessary for differential diagnosis[2]

REFERENCES

1. Jarvis C. *Physical Examination and Health Assessment.* 5th ed. St. Louis, MO: Saunders-Elsevier; 2008.
2. Kreis ME, Edler v. Koch F, Jauch KW, Friese K. The differential diagnosis of right lower quadrant pain. *Dtsch Arztebl.* 2007;104(45):A3114–3121. http://aerzteblatt.lnsdata.de/pdf/DI/104/45/a3114e.pdf. Accessed on March 19, 2010.

ABDOMEN

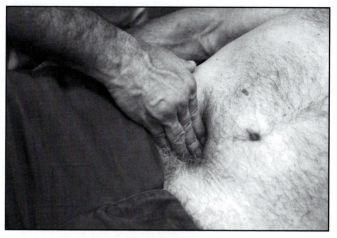

FIGURE 3-13. REBOUND TENDERNESS.

ABDOMEN

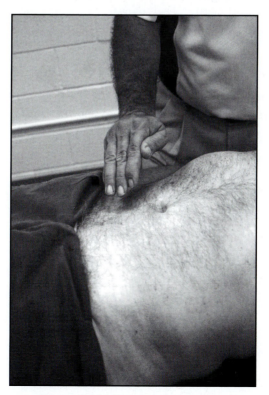

FIGURE 3-14. REBOUND TENDERNESS.

ABDOMEN

MURPHY'S SIGN

TEST POSITION

- Supine on exam table, head on pillow, arms at sides, knees bent to 90° or supported by pillows (for relaxation) with examiner standing at right side

ACTION[1]

- Client exhales
- Hook 4 fingers of the right hand under the costal margin of the RUQ to feel for the liver
- Client inhales deeply

NORMAL FINDINGS

- No pain and completion of respiratory cycle

POSITIVE FINDINGS

- Sharp pain with inspiration, with client often unable to complete a deep inspiration; may indicate inflammation of the gall bladder

SPECIAL CONSIDERATIONS

- Sensitivity = 97.2%; specificity = 48.3%
- Positive predictive value = 70%, and the negative predictive value = 93.3%[2]

REFERENCES

1. Jarvis C. *Physical Examination and Health Assessment.* 5th ed. St. Louis, MO: Saunders-Elsevier; 2008.
2. Urbano FL, Carroll MB. Murphy's sign of cholecystitis. *Hospital Physician.* 2000;11:51-52,70. http://www.turner-white.com/pdf/hp_nov00_murphy.pdf. Accessed on March 19, 2010.

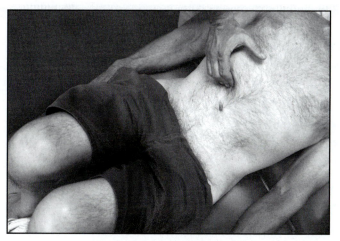

FIGURE 3-15. MURPHY'S SIGN.

Iliopsoas Muscle Test for Appendicitis

Test Position

- Supine on exam table, head on pillow, arms at sides with examiner standing on the right side of the client with left hand above the client's right knee

Action

- Flex right hip to 90° against light resistance; client then turns to left lateral decubitus position to extend right leg[1]

Normal Findings

- No pain

Positive Findings

- Pain in the LRQ with right knee flexion or extension

Special Consideration

- Specificity = .95; sensitivity = .16[2]

References

1. Jarvis C. *Physical Examination and Health Assessment.* 5th ed. St. Louis, MO: Saunders-Elsevier; 2008.
2. Wagner JM, McKinney WP, Carpenter JL. Does this patient have appendicitis? *JAMA.* 1996;276:1589-1594.

ABDOMEN

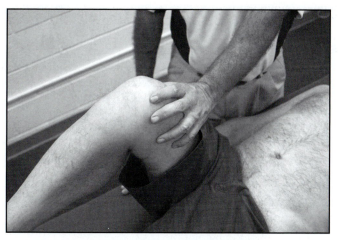

FIGURE 3-16. ILIOPSOAS TEST POSITION 1.

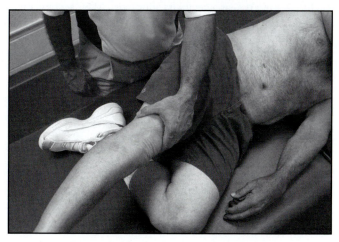

FIGURE 3-17. ILIOPSOAS TEST POSITION 2.

ABDOMEN

OBTURATOR MUSCLE TEST FOR APPENDICITIS

TEST POSITION
- Supine, head on pillow, arms at side, knees extended with examiner standing on the right side of the client

ACTION
- Examiner passively abducts the right hip to 45° and the knee to 90° while internally rotating the hip

NORMAL FINDINGS
- No pain

POSITIVE FINDINGS
- Pain in the LRQ but not the LLQ

SPECIAL CONSIDERATION
- No sensitivity or specificity findings. May accompany other signs and symptoms of appendicitis, such as RLQ pain, rigidity, and migration of pain from umbilicus[1-3]

REFERENCES
1. Jarvis C. *Physical Examination and Health Assessment.* 5th ed. St. Louis, MO: Saunders-Elsevier; 2008.
2. Wagner JM, McKinney WP, Carpenter JL. Does this patient have appendicitis? *JAMA.* 1996;276:1589-1594.
3. Orient JM. *Sapira's Art & Science of Bedside Diagnosis.* 3rd ed. Philadelphia, PA: Lippincott Williams & Wilkins; 2005:451.

ABDOMEN

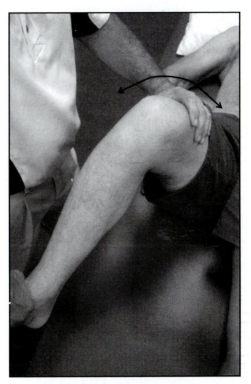

FIGURE 3-18. OBTURATOR TEST.

ASSESSMENT OF DIASTASIS RECTI

TEST POSITION
- Supine on exam table, head on pillow, arms at sides, knees bent to 90° or supported by pillows (for relaxation) with examiner standing at right side

ACTION
- With fingertips held vertically, palpate rectus abdominis separation 2 inches above and 2 inches below umbilicus, while client raises head and shoulder blades off of examination table

NORMAL FINDINGS
- <1 finger width separation between left and right rectus abdominis muscle[1]

POSITIVE FINDINGS
- >2 finger or 2-cm separation between left and right rectus abdominis[1]

SPECIAL CONSIDERATION
- Minor separations may be improved through exercise

REFERENCE
1. Donnelly C. Back pain after baby: the missing link. http://www.bodyinsight101.com/blog/index.php?s=diastasis+recti. Accessed on March 19, 2010.

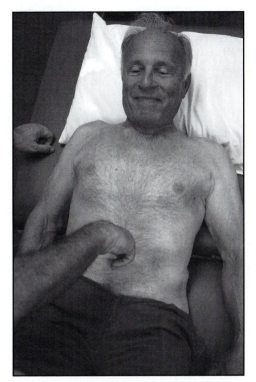

FIGURE 3-19. PALPATION OF DIASTASIS RECTI.

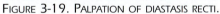

Section

FOUR

Examination of the Peripheral Vascular System

PERIPHERAL VASCULAR HISTORY: DIFFERENTIAL DIAGNOSIS FOR ARTERIAL AND VENOUS DISEASES

TEST POSITION

- Long sitting on plinth or with feet in dependent position

ACTION

- Ask questions related to symptoms
- Observe and examine extremities for signs of arterial or venous disease
- Compare one limb to the other, as well as proximal and distal components of each leg/foot

NORMAL FINDINGS

- Asymptomatic extremities at rest, with elevation/dependency and activity

POSITIVE FINDINGS

See Table 4-1 on the following page.

SPECIAL CONSIDERATIONS

- Chronic venous disorders include varicose veins or valvular incompetence
- Peripheral vascular disease (PVD) or peripheral arterial disease (PAD) refer to arteries that have atherosclerotic plaque build-up
- PAD affects 15% to 20% of Americans over 65 years of age[1]
- Individuals with PAD symptoms likely have similar subclinical disease in their coronary arteries, carotid, and cerebrovascular systems
- When posterior tibial and dorsalis pedis pulses are both absent, there is a high probability the patient has PAD[2]
- Bruits represent blood flow disturbance at the stenotic site[1]

REFERENCES

1. Creager MA, Libby P. Peripheral arterial diseases. In: Libby P, Bonow RO, Mann DL, Zipes DP, eds. *Braunwald's Heart Disease: A Textbook of Cardiovascular Medicine*. 8th ed. Philadelphia, PA: Saunders Co; 2008:1495.
2. Stoffers HE, Kester AD, Kaiser V, Rinkens PE, Knottnerus JA. Diagnostic value of signs and symptoms associated with peripheral arterial occlusive disease seen in general practice: a multivariable approach. *Med Decis Making*. 1997;17:61-70.

O'Connell DG, O'Connell JK, Hinman MR.
Special Tests of the Cardiopulmonary, Vascular and Gastrointestinal Systems (pp 130-196).
© 2011 SLACK Incorporated

PERIPHERAL
VASCULAR SYSTEM

Table 4-1

DIFFERENCES BETWEEN ARTERIAL AND VENOUS DISORDERS

Descriptor	Venous Disorders	Arterial Disorders
Symptoms	Aching, burning, cramping, fatigue while standing, heaviness, night cramping, swelling, throbbing	Aching or cramping that is predictable with activity and elevation
Elevation	Lessens symptoms	Worsens symptoms, dependency improves symptoms[1]
Walking exercise	Lessens symptoms	Aching begins at specific time/distance, goes away with rest, returns with exercise[1]
Limb size	Swollen in chronic disease	Decreased due to muscle wasting
Muscle mass	Normal	Reduced[1]
Elevation	Lessens symptoms	Worsens symptoms
Skin temperature	May be warm with infection, phlebitis	Cool to touch[1]
Skin color	Hyperpigmented (bluish-brown), often superior to medial malleolus	Cyanotic or pale, dependent rubor[1]
Skin (other)	Chronic cellulitis, dermatitis, ulceration	Reduced hair; thick/brittle toenails; tight, shiny skin[1]
Pulses	May be difficult to palpate 2° to edema	May be decreased or absent; bruits may be present[1]
Ulcers	Often near medial malleolus, very irregular border, often with pink base[1]	Pale base, discrete circumscribed borders, found at high-pressure sites, such as the heel or tips of toes[1]

Adapted from Creager MA, Libby P. Peripheral arterial diseases. In: Libby P, Bonow RO, Mann DL, Zipes DP, eds. *Braunwald's Heart Disease: A Textbook of Cardiovascular Medicine.* 8th ed. Philadelphia, PA: Saunders Co; 2008:1495 and Stoffers HE, Kester AD, Kaiser V, Rinkens PE, Knottnerus JA. Diagnostic value of signs and symptoms associated with peripheral arterial occlusive disease seen in general practice: a multivariable approach. *Med Decis Making.* 1997;17:61-70.

PERIPHERAL VASCULAR SYSTEM

ASSESSING THE INTEGUMENTARY SYSTEM
FOR SKIN CANCER

TEST POSITION

- Supine, seated, or standing

ACTION

- As body parts are exposed for examination, observe and assess using the "ABCD" rubric[1] for melanomas

Table 4-2

IDENTIFYING SKIN LESIONS
REQUIRING FURTHER EVALUATION

A	Asymmetrical	Lesion halves do not look alike
B	Borders	Irregular edges are notched, ragged, or blurred
C	Color	Multicolored pigmentation (black, tan, brown)
D	Diameter	>6 mm, or about the size of a pencil eraser
E[2]	Evolving	Changes in A to D, or new symptoms such as bleeding, itching, crusting

Adapted from Cancer Facts & Figures 2008. American Cancer Society, Inc. http://www.cancer.org/downloads/STT/2008CAFFfinalsecured.pdf. Accessed March 19, 2010.

- Obtain pertinent history of changes in size, shape, color of skin lesion, or the appearance of a new growth on skin[1,2]

NORMAL FINDINGS

- Unchanging lesions that do not meet the criteria above

ABNORMAL FINDINGS[1]

- Lesions changing for >30 days are suspicious
- Moles that grow, or a new growth on skin
- Lesions that are not small, symmetrical, with a singular color, and regular borders
- Growths that are flat, firm, and pale, or small, raised, pink, or red; translucent shiny areas that bleed following minor injury are suggestive of basal cell carcinoma

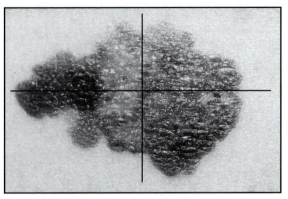

FIGURE 4-1. PHOTOGRAPH OF MELANOMA. (PHOTO
COURTESY OF NATIONAL CANCER INSTITUTE.)

- Growing lumps often with a rough surface, or flat, slow-growing, reddish patches are suggestive of squamous cell carcinoma
- Sores that do not heal

SPECIAL CONSIDERATIONS[1]

- Initiate prevention strategies in childhood
- Limit sun exposure to before 10 AM and after 4 PM
- Use SPF >15, and wear hats, long sleeves, and pants
- Adults should engage in annual skin check-ups
- 80% of melanomas are diagnosed when 5-year survival rate is 99%

REFERENCES

1. Cancer Facts & Figures 2008. American Cancer Society, Inc. http://www.cancer.org/downloads/STT/2008CAFFfinalsecured.pdf. Accessed March 19, 2010.
2. Self examination. Skin Cancer Foundation. http://www.skincancer.org/Self-Examination/. Accessed March 19, 2010.

PERIPHERAL
VASCULAR SYSTEM

SKIN TURGOR

TEST POSITION
- Relaxed, seated

ACTION
- Use thumb and index finger to grasp skin (few seconds) on dorsum of hand, lower arm, or abdomen (child) to briefly form a tent, then release

NORMAL FINDINGS
- Rapid snap of skin to normal position

POSITIVE FINDINGS
- Decreased turgor noted when skin remains tented

SPECIAL CONSIDERATIONS
- Decreased turgor is a late sign of dehydration occurring in moderate to severe dehydration
- Fluid loss of 5%, 10%, and 15% is considered to be mild, moderate, and severe dehydration, respectively

PERIPHERAL
VASCULAR SYSTEM

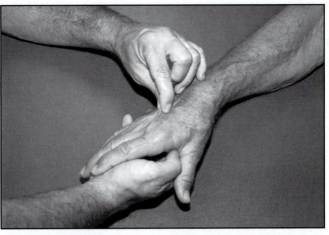

FIGURE 4-2. ASSESSING TURGOR.

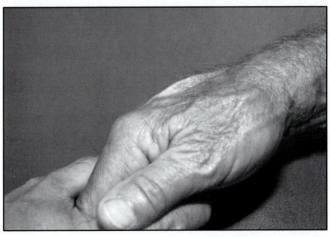

FIGURE 4-3. TENTING.

PERIPHERAL
VASCULAR SYSTEM

SKIN TEMPERATURE

TEST POSITION

- Supine examination of the lower extremities, although self-assessment of foot temperature can be done with infrared skin thermography[1]

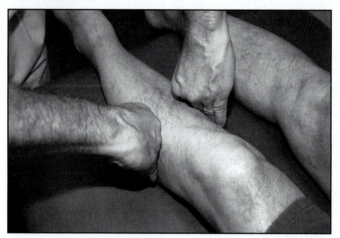

FIGURE 4-4. ASSESSING SKIN TEMPERATURE WITH DORSAL HANDS.

ACTION

- Test skin temperature with dorsal phalanges starting on the proximal lower leg moving distally toward the toes

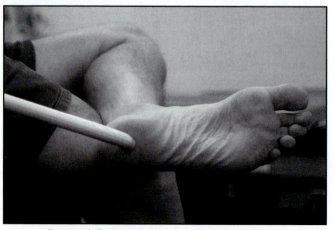

FIGURE 4-5. ASSESSING SKIN TEMPERATURE WITH
THERMOMETRY PROBE.

- Alternatively, dermal thermometry can be used on 6 sites on the dorsal surface of each foot[2] comparing right vs left

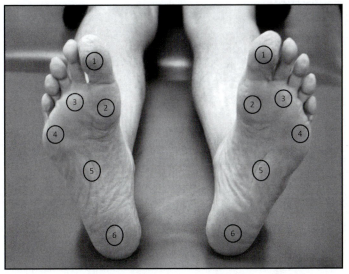

FIGURE 4-6. THERMOMETRY SITES.

NORMAL FINDINGS

- Skin temperature is 82°F to 90°F depending on room temperature[2]
- Proximal to distal symmetric, bilateral decrease in temperature[2]
- Interlimb dermal thermography difference ≤4°F in those with diabetes[1]

POSITIVE FINDINGS

- Lower or higher than normal skin temperatures via palpation[2]
- Unilateral difference in skin temperature via palpation[2]
- In diabetes, temperature differences of >4°F between extremities usually triggers more intensive medical care[1]

SPECIAL CONSIDERATIONS

- Warm extremities suggest infection, inflammatory processes, (including vasculitis or phlebitis), or venous insufficiency, venous stasis, or hyperemia suggest venous disease[2]
- Cool extremities suggest ischemia[2] and correlate with infrared findings[3]

- Foot temperature differences are significantly greater in those that ulcerate than in those that do not ulcerate[1]

REFERENCES

1. Armstrong DG, Holtz-Neiderer K, Wendel C, Mohler MJ, Kimbriel HR, Lavery LA. Skin temperature monitoring reduces the risk of diabetic foot ulceration in high-risk patients. *Am J Med.* 2007;120:1042-1046.

2. Nelson JP. The vascular history and physical examination. *Clin Pod Med Surg.* 1992;9:1-13.

3. Boyko EJ, Ahroni JH, Davignon D, Stensel V, Prigeon RL, Smith DG. Diagnostic utility of the history and physical examination for peripheral vascular disease among patients with diabetes mellitus. *J Clin Epidemiol.* 1997;50:659-668.

PERIPHERAL VASCULAR SYSTEM

FIGURE-OF-EIGHT METHODS FOR MEASURING LIMB EDEMA

TEST POSITIONS

- Foot: Long sitting with foot extending over edge of table
- Ankle: In neutral, dorsiflexed position
- Hand: Seated with forearm resting pronated with hand extending over edge of table
- Wrist: Held in a neutral position with fingers adducted and extended

ACTION (FOR MEASURING THE FOOT)[1]

- Using a standard, flexible tape measure, start midway between the tibialis anterior tendon and the lateral malleolus and draw the tape measure medially across the instep distal to the navicular tuberosity
- Pull across the arch to the base of the 5th metatarsal, diagonally across the dorsum of the foot to the medial malleolus, across the Achilles tendon to the lateral malleolus, and back to the starting point
- Record average of 3 measurements

ACTION (FOR MEASURING THE HAND)[2]

- Using a standard, flexible tape measure, start at the distal aspect of the ulnar styloid process and draw the tape measure across the ventral surface of the wrist to the radial styloid, then diagonally across the dorsum of the hand to the 5th metacarpophalangeal (MCP) joint, then across the palm to the 2nd MCP joint, then diagonally across the dorsum of the hand back to the ulnar styloid
- Record average of 3 measurements

SPECIAL CONSIDERATIONS/COMMENTS

- High correlations (r) for figure-of-eight and volumetric measures r = 92 to 95: hand, r = 88 to 96: foot[2-9]
- Intra- and interrater reliability range from 0.98 to 0.99 for both measurements[2-9]
- Minimal detectable change for the foot is approximately 1 cm[9]

REFERENCES

1. Esterson PS. Measurement of ankle joint swelling using a figure of 8. *J Orthop Sports Phys Ther.* 1979;1:51-52.

2. Pellecchia GL. Figure-of-eight method of measuring hand size: reliability and concurrent validity. *J Hand Ther.* 2003;16:300-304.

3. Maihafer GC, Llewellyn MA, Pillar WJ Jr, Scott KL, Marino DM, Bond RM. A comparison of figure-of-eight method and water volumetry in measurement of hand and wrist size. *J Hand Ther.* 2003;16:305-310.

4. Leard JS, Breglio L, Fraga L, et al. Reliability and concurrent validity of the figure-of-eight method of measuring hand size in patient with hand pathology. *J Orthop Sport Phys Ther.* 2004;34:335-340.

5. Tatro-Adams D, McGann SF, Carbone W. Reliability of the figure-of-eight method of ankle measurement. *J Orthop Sports Phys Ther.* 1995;22:161-163.

6. Petersen EJ, Irish SM, Lyons CL, et al. Reliability of water volumetry and the figure of eight method on subjects with ankle joint swelling. *J Orthop Sports Phys Ther.* 1999;29:609-615.

7. Mawdsley RH, Hoy DK, Erwin PM. Criterion-related validity of the figure-of-eight method of measuring ankle edema. *J Orthop Sports Phys Ther.* 2000;30:149-153.

8. Friends J, Augustine E, Danoff J. A comparison of different assessment techniques for measuring foot and ankle volume in healthy adults. *J Am Podiatr Med Assoc.* 2008;98:85-94.

9. Rohner-Spengler M, Mannion AF, Babst R. Reliability and minimal detectable change for the figure-of-eight method of measurement of ankle edema. *J Orthop Sports Phys Ther.* 2007;37:199-205.

PERIPHERAL
VASCULAR SYSTEM

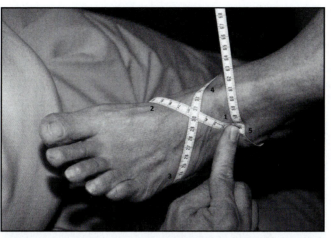

FIGURE 4-7. FIGURE-OF-EIGHT FOOT.

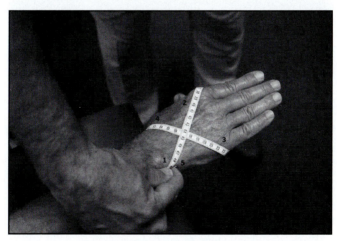

FIGURE 4-8. FIGURE-OF-EIGHT HAND.

Volumetric Measures of Limb Edema (Water Displacement Method)

Test Positions

- Foot: Seated in chair, foot placed inside volumeter with toes facing spout end, heel positioned firmly on the bottom

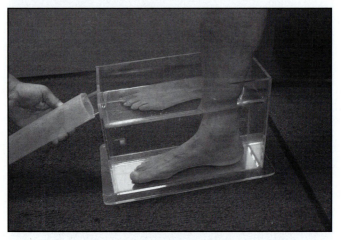

FIGURE 4-9. VOLUMETRIC ASSESSMENT OF FOOT.

- Hand: Standing or seated, arm placed inside volumeter with palm turned inward, thumb pointing toward the spout
  - ✧ 3rd and 4th fingers web space rest on dowel; if no dowel is used, tip of 3rd finger should rest on the bottom of volumeter (see Figure 4-10 on following page)

Action

- Place plexiglas volumeter on floor or table and fill with tepid water until the water overflow stops flowing out of the spout
- Slowly immerse test limb and catch overflow of displaced water in graduated cylinder, measuring volume

Special Considerations

- Accuracy of volumetry is <1% and detectable change is 10 mL[1]
- Volumetric measurements are highly reproducible with ICCs of 0.99[1-5]

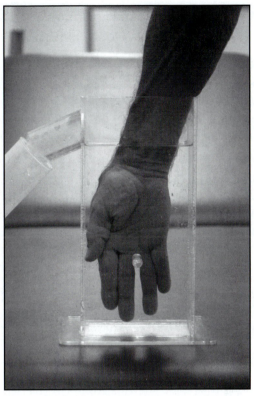

FIGURE 4-10. VOLUMETRIC ASSESSMENT OF HAND.

REFERENCES

1. Boland R, Adams R. Development and evaluation of a precision forearm and hand volumeter and measuring cylinder. *J Hand Ther.* 1996;9:349-358.

2. Pellecchia GL. Figure-of-eight method of measuring hand size: reliability and concurrent validity. *J Hand Ther.* 2003;16:300-304.

3. Petersen EJ, Irish SM, Lyons CL, et al. Reliability of water volumetry and the figure of eight method on subjects with ankle joint swelling. *J Orthop Sports Phys Ther.* 1999;29:609-615.

4. Friends J, Augustine E, Danoff J. A comparison of different assessment techniques for measuring foot and ankle volume in healthy adults. *J Am Podiatr Med Assoc.* 2008;98:85-94.

5. Karges JR, Mark BE, Stikeleather SJ, Worrell TW. Concurrent validity of upper-extremity volume estimates: comparison of calculated volume derived from girth measurements and water displacement volume. *Phys Ther.* 2003;83:134-145.

GIRTH MEASUREMENTS AND ESTIMATED LIMB SEGMENT VOLUME

TEST POSITIONS

- Lower extremity: Standing or supine-leg extended and foot propped up on a stool to avoid contact with the tabletop
- Upper extremity: Seated with the arm horizontally abducted, hand supported on stable object (back of chair or tabletop)

ACTION: GIRTH MEASUREMENTS

- Lower extremity: Record limb circumference at knee joint line or tibial tubercle and repeat measurement at 10-cm (1.5-in) intervals distal and proximal, according to the extent of the edema
- Upper extremity: Select appropriate landmark (MCP joints or styloid processes), measure, and record limb circumference there and at 10-cm intervals to axilla (or along extent of the edema)

ACTION: CALCULATE VOLUME USING FRUSTUM (TRUNCATED CONE) FORMULA

- Obtain/record length between proximal and distal girth measurements
- Estimate volume (V) of the edematous segment

$$V = h\ (C_1{}^2 + C_1 C_2 + C_2{}^2)\ /\ 12\pi$$

  where C_1 and C_2 are the circumferences at the ends of the segment and h is the distance between them
- Estimate volume of entire limb by adding volumes of multiple segments

SPECIAL CONSIDERATIONS

- Intra- and interrater reliability of lower extremity girth measurements are r = 0.82 to 1.00 and 0.72 to 0.97, respectively[1,2]
- Reliability of upper extremity girth measurements are r = 0.97 to 0.99[3-5]
- Estimated volumetric measurements are highly reproducible and correlate well (r = 0.96 to 0.99) with water displacement[3]
- Girth and volumetric measurements are not equivalent and cannot be used interchangeably

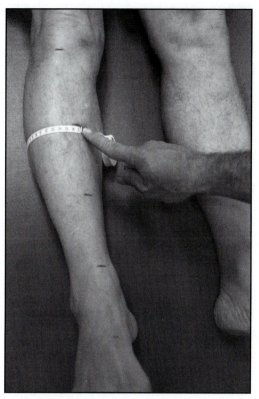

FIGURE 4-11. GIRTH ASSESSMENT OF LEG.

PERIPHERAL
VASCULAR SYSTEM

REFERENCES

1. Whitney SL, Mattocks I, Irrgang JJ, et al. Reliability of lower extremity girth measurements and right- and left-side differences. *J Sport Rehabil.* 1995;4:108-115.

2. Soderberg FL, Ballantyne BT, Kestel LL. Reliability of lower extremity girth measurements after anterior cruciate ligament reconstruction. *Physiother Res Int.* 1996;1:7-16.

3. Sander AP, Hajer NM, Hemenway K, Miller AC. Upper-extremity volume measurements in women with lymphedema: a comparison of measurements obtained via water displacement with geometrically determined volume. *Phys Ther.* 2002;82:1201-1212.

4. Karges JR, Mark BE, Stikeleather SJ, Worrell TW. Concurrent validity of upper-extremity volume estimates: comparison of calculated volume derived from girth measurements and water displacement volume. *Phys Ther.* 2003;83:134-145.

PERIPHERAL
VASCULAR SYSTEM

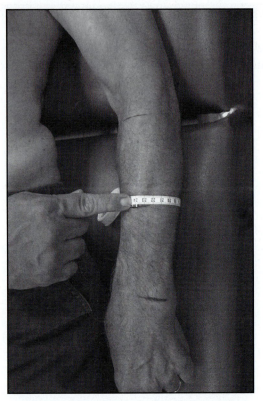

FIGURE 4-12. GIRTH ASSESSMENT OF ARM.

5. Taylor R, Jayasinghe UW, Koelmeyer L, Ung O, Boyages J. Reliability and validity of arm volume measurements for assessment of lymphedema. *Phys Ther.* 2006;86:205-214.

CAPILLARY REFILL TIME TEST (CRTT)

TEST POSITION

- Seated with hands near heart level for distal finger measurement
- Long-sitting position for distal great toe measurement

ACTION

- Remove nail polish
- Depress nail beds for 5 seconds so they blanch (turn white)
- Time and note when color returns

NORMAL FINDINGS

- Capillary refill (distal finger) <3 seconds is most often noted as normal[1]
- Capillary refill (distal great toe) ≤5 sec (diabetic sample)[2,3]

POSITIVE FINDINGS

- Capillary refill (distal finger) ≥3 seconds[1]
- Capillaries refill (distal great toe) >5 seconds[1] (diabetic sample)[2,3]

SPECIAL CONSIDERATIONS

- Median and 95th percentile values in 1000 normal adults were 1.9 sec and 3.5 sec respectively[4]
- Good intratester reliability (ICC = 0.72); variable intertester reliability (ICC range = 0.12-0.81)[5]
- CRTT predicts less than 40% of the variance in laser Doppler flowmetry measures and does not discriminate between those with and without peripheral arterial disease or impaired healing[4]
- In healthy adult subjects, age, gender, ambient temperature, and patient temperature explained only 8% of the observed variance but were significant predictors of CRRT[4]
- Positive findings may suggest peripheral vascular disease, decreased cardiac output, or ineffective oxygenation secondary to pulmonary or blood disorder
- Low body temperature or hypothermia, vasoconstriction due to nicotine, peripheral edema, and anemia can also cause poor capillary refill

PERIPHERAL VASCULAR SYSTEM

- A reliable test when performed by experienced clinicians, but the test has variable interrater reliability, limited predictability, and limited normative standards

REFERENCES

1. Jarvis C. *Physical Examination and Health Assessment.* 5th ed. St. Louis, MO: Saunders-Elsevier; 2008:537.

2. Boyko EJ, Ahroni JH, Davignon D, Stensel V, Prigeon RL, Smith DG. Diagnostic utility of the history and physical examination for peripheral vascular disease among patients with diabetes mellitus. *J Clin. Epidemiol.* 1997;50:659-668.

3. Abramson DI. *Circulatory Problems in Podiatry.* Basal, Switzerland: Karger; 1985:33.

4. Anderson B, Kelly AM, Kerr D, Clooney M, Jolley D. Impact of patient and environmental factors on capillary refill time in adults. *Am J Emerg Med.* 2008; 26:62-65.

5. Klupp NL, Keena AM. An evaluation of the reliability and validity of capillary refill time test. *The Foot.* 2007:17;15-20.

PERIPHERAL VASCULAR SYSTEM

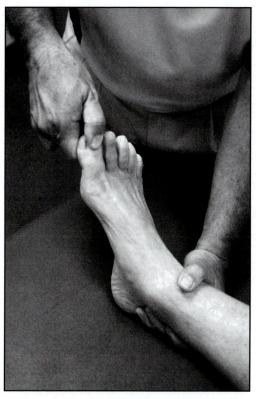

FIGURE 4-13. CAPILLARY REFILL OF GREAT TOE.

ELEVATION PALLOR

TEST POSITION
- Supine

ACTION
- Elevate legs to 60° and hold in place
- Examine color of soles of feet

FINDINGS[1]

Table 4-3		
ELEVATION PALLOR TEST		
Grade	*Coloration*	*Duration*
0	No pallor	in 60 sec
1+	Pallor	in 60 sec
2+	Pallor	31-60 sec
3+	Pallor	< 30 sec
4+	Pallor	0 sec, feet level with heart

Adapted from Spittel JA. Recognition and management of chronic atherosclerotic occlusive peripheral arterial disease. *Mod Concepts Cardivas Disease.* 1981;50:19-23.

SPECIAL CONSIDERATIONS
- Pale discoloration suggests peripheral arterial occlusion[1-3]
- With extremities at heart level, pooled blood masks the arterial flow
- Elevation of extremities increases venous drainage, allowing for an accurate assessment of the degree of arterial flow

REFERENCES
1. Spittel JA. Recognition and management of chronic atherosclerotic occlusive peripheral arterial disease. *Mod Concepts Cardivas Disease.* 1981;50:19-23.
2. Halloran DT, Blume PA, Palladino MG, Sumpio BE. How to perform a thorough vascular exam. *Podiatry Today.* http://www.podiatrytoday.com/article/7074. Accessed March 25, 2010.
3. Sumpio BE, Lee T, Blume PA. Vascular evaluation and arterial reconstruction of the diabetic foot. *Clin Podiatr Med Surg.* 2003;20:689-708.

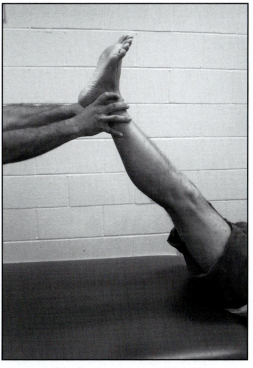

FIGURE 4-14. ELEVATION PALLOR LATERAL VIEW.

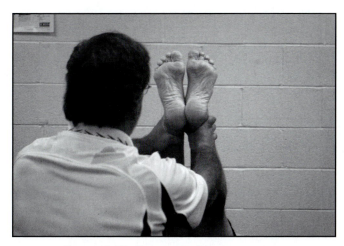

FIGURE 4-15. ELEVATION PALLOR LONG VIEW.

PERIPHERAL
VASCULAR SYSTEM

STOOP TEST

TEST POSITION
- Standing and stooping forward or sitting

ACTION
- Obtain history of pain associated with movement
- Client is asked to walk briskly
- If pain occurs, client is asked to continue walking
- Note if client stoops forward while walking
  - ✧ Forward stooping may cause pain relief
- If so, ask client to stand upright to see if pain returns
- If pain returns, client is asked to sit and stoop forward in chair
  - ✧ Determine if forward stooping relieves pain

NORMAL FINDINGS
- No pain in low back, buttocks, or legs upon walking[1]

POSITIVE FINDINGS
- Pain relief upon forward stooping while walking or in sitting[1]

SPECIAL CONSIDERATIONS
- Pain relief with forward stooping suggests intermittent cauda equina compression syndrome rather than intermittent claudication
- Altered reflexes, decreased strength, decreased sensation, and altered bowel or bladder function should prompt seeking further medical attention
- There is a paucity of research on this test

REFERENCE
1. Dyck P. The stoop-test in lumbar entrapment radiculopathy. *Spine.* 1979;4:89-92.

PERIPHERAL VASCULAR SYSTEM

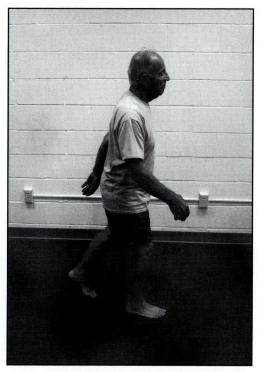

FIGURE 4-16. WALKING.

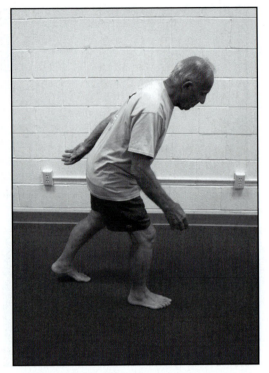

FIGURE 4-17. WALKING WITH STOOPING.

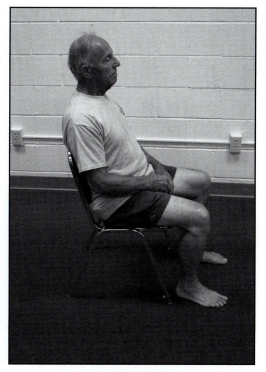

FIGURE 4-18. SITTING.

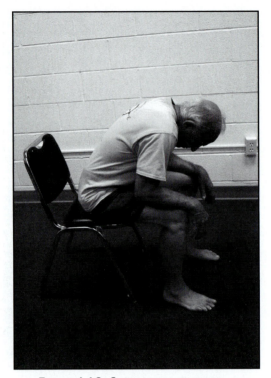

FIGURE 4-19. SITTING WITH STOOPING.

TREADMILL TIME TO CLAUDICATION

TEST POSITION

- Walking on a calibrated treadmill

ACTION

- Measure ankle brachial index (ABI) before, within 1 minute of test cessation, and then every minute in supine recovery until ABI returns to preexercise levels[1]
- Protocol #1: Constant grade = 12%, increase speed 1.5 or 2.0 mph
- Protocol #2: Constant speed = 2 mph, increase grade 2%, every 2 minutes
- Use Claudication Scale during test[2]

Table 4-4

TREADMILL TIME TO CLAUDICATION

Rating	Pain/Discomfort Level	Description
1	Minimal	Barely noticeable pain
2	Moderate	Attention can be diverted
3	Intense	Attention cannot be diverted
4	Excruciating, unbearable	Worst pain ever experienced

Adapted from American College of Sports Medicine. *ACSM Guidelines for Exercise Testing and Exercise Prescription.* Baltimore, MD: Lippincott Williams & Wilkins; 2010.

- Record when claudication begins, initial claudication distance (ICD), or time and terminate test when the patient reaches a maximal level of claudication pain (absolute claudication distance [ACD]) or time[1,3]
- Record any other ischemic symptoms[1,3]

NORMAL FINDINGS

- No claudication pain during or following walking

POSITIVE FINDINGS

- Postexercise decrease in ABI ≥25% when walking is limited by claudication is diagnostic for PAD[4]

PERIPHERAL VASCULAR SYSTEM

SPECIAL CONSIDERATION

- Supervised rehabilitative walking programs of 30 to 45 minutes per session, 3 times per week for a minimum of 12 weeks[1] to 6 months[2] have been shown to increase distance to onset of claudication pain, distance to maximal claudication pain, and total distance walked[5,6]
- ACD should be used as the resting point between walking intervals

REFERENCES

1. Hirsh AT, Haskal ZJ, Hertzer NR, et al. ACC/AHA 2005 practice guidelines for the management of patients with peripheral arterial disease (lower extremity, renal, mesenteric, and abdominal aortic): a collaborative report from the American Association for Vascular Surgery/Society for Vascular Surgery, Society for Cardiovascular Angiography and Interventions, Society for Vascular Medicine and Biology, Society of Interventional Radiology, and the ACC/AHA Task Force on Practice Guidelines (Writing Committee to Develop Guidelines for the Management of Patients With Peripheral Arterial Disease): endorsed by the American Association of Cardiovascular and Pulmonary Rehabilitation; National Heart, Lung, and Blood Institute; Society for Vascular Nursing; TransAtlantic Inter-Society Consensus; and Vascular Disease Foundation. *Circulation.* 2006;113:e463-e654.

2. American College of Sports Medicine. *ACSM Guidelines for Exercise Testing and Exercise Prescription.* Baltimore, MD: Lippincott Williams & Wilkins; 2010.

3. Hiatt WR, Hirsch AT, Regensteiner JG, et al. Clinical trials for claudication: assessment of exercise performance, functional status, and clinical end points. *Circulation.* 1995;92:614-621.

4. Creager MA, Libby P. Peripheral arterial diseases. In: Libby P, Bonow RO, Mann DL, Zipes DP, eds. *Braunwald's Heart Disease: A Textbook of Cardiovascular Medicine.* 8th ed. Philadelphia, PA: Saunders Co; 2008.

5. Gardner AW, Katzel LI, Sorkin JD, et al. Improved functional outcomes following exercise rehabilitation in patients with intermittent claudication. *J Gerontol A Biol Sci Med Sci.* 2000;55:M570-M577.

6. Gardner AW, Poehlman ET. Exercise rehabilitation programs for the treatment of claudication pain: a meta-analysis. *JAMA.* 1995;274:975-980.

PERIPHERAL
VASCULAR SYSTEM

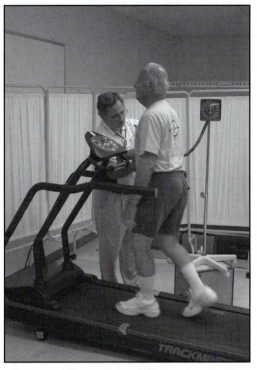

FIGURE 4-20. TREADMILL CLAUDICATION TEST.

ACTIVE PEDAL PLANTARFLEXION (APP) INTERMITTENT CLAUDICATION TEST

TEST POSITION

- Standing for pedal plantarflexion test; supine for ABI measurement

ACTION

- ABI measured prior to and within 1 minute following the test
- Stand facing wall, knees fully extended, elbows flexed—slightly less than 90° with fingertips touching wall for balance
- Perform up to 50 consecutive symptom-limited repetitions of plantar flexion[1]
- Observe for quality of plantar flexion and record time to complete test

NORMAL FINDINGS

- ≥43±10 repetitions in those with known/suspected peripheral arterial disease

POSITIVE FINDINGS

- <33 repetitions and/or pain severe enough to cause test cessation

SPECIAL CONSIDERATIONS

- Study of 100 legs with known or suspected peripheral arterial disease revealed strong correlations between (r = 0.77 to 0.90) those with less severe disease (ABI >0.8) and those with more significant disease (ABI ≤0.8)[1]
- Posttest ABI measurements for treadmill and APP tests were not significantly different[1]
- The APP test is a simple, safe, accurate, and objective noninvasive evaluative tool for those with known or suspected peripheral arterial disease[1]

REFERENCE

1. McPhail IR, Spittell PC, Weston SA, Bailey KR. Intermittent claudication: an objective office-based assessment. *J Am Coll Cardiol.* 2001;37:1381-1385.

PERIPHERAL VASCULAR SYSTEM

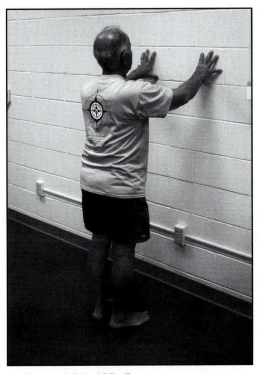

FIGURE 4-21. APP: FLAT-FOOTED STANCE.

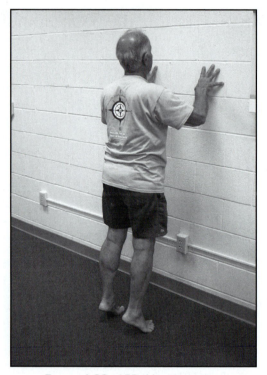

FIGURE 4-22. APP: HEELS RAISED.

ALLEN'S TEST FOR HAND CIRCULATION

TEST POSITION
- Seated or standing

ACTION
- Client opens and closes hand quickly several times before making tight fist
- Examiner places thumbs over radial and ulnar arteries at styloid level
- Client open hands so palm is visible
- Examiner removes thumb pressure from one artery and refilling assessed
- Procedure repeated for remaining artery
- Compare both hands

NORMAL FINDINGS
- Refilling of both radial and ulnar arteries

POSITIVE FINDINGS
- Palm remains pale when vessel is released

SPECIAL CONSIDERATION
- Test determines major arterial supply to the hand

REFERENCE
1. Magee DJ. *Orthopedic Physical Assessment.* 5th ed. St. Louis, MO: Saunders; 2008.

PERIPHERAL VASCULAR SYSTEM

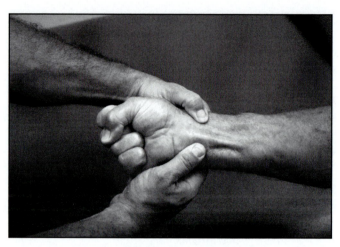

FIGURE 4-23. CLOSED FIST.

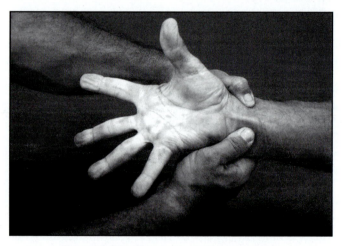

FIGURE 4-24. OPEN HAND WITH BLANCHING.

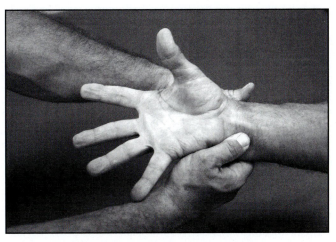

FIGURE 4-25. RADIAL ARTERY RELEASED.

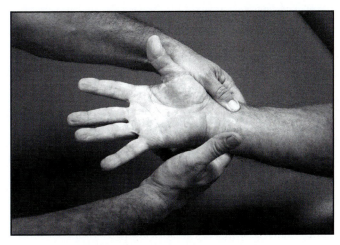

FIGURE 4-26. ULNAR ARTERY RELEASED.

VERTEBRAL ARTERY TEST

TEST POSITION

- Supine, eyes open

ACTION

- Obtain recent history related to symptoms such as dizziness, diplopia, dysphasia, dysarthria, drop attacks, nausea, and nystagmus[1]
- Passively position head/neck into extension, then side bending, and finally lateral rotation to the same side[2]
- Hold each position for 10 to 30 seconds[2]
- Stop test if symptoms occur and avoid cervical mobilization/manipulation
- Negative test, return head/neck to neutral, then test contralateral side

NORMAL FINDINGS

- No signs or symptoms of intolerance

POSITIVE FINDINGS

- Nystagmus, dizziness, light-headedness, nausea

SPECIAL CONSIDERATIONS

- Positive tests should be repeated on a different day
- Refer for further testing with 2 positive test results
- The vertebral artery test has zero sensitivity and high specificity but is commonly performed for medical-legal purposes[2]

REFERENCES

1. Cook CE, Hegedus EJ. *Orthopedic Physical Examination Tests: An Evidence-Based Approach.* Upper Saddle River, NJ: Pearson Prentice Hall; 2008.
2. Magee DJ. *Orthopedic Physical Assessment.* 5th ed. St. Louis, MO: Saunders; 2008.

PERIPHERAL
VASCULAR SYSTEM

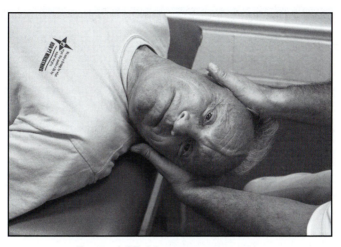

FIGURE 4-27. VERTEBRAL ARTERY TEST.

ROOS TEST FOR
THORACIC OUTLET SYNDROME (TOS)

TEST POSITION
- Seated, shoulders abducted 90° slightly behind frontal plane, elbows flexed 90°[1]

ACTION
- Open and close hands slowly for 3 minutes

NORMAL FINDINGS
- Completion of 3-minute test with minor fatigue

POSITIVE FINDINGS
- Inability to maintain position
- Ischemic pain, heaviness, profound arm weakness, numbness, or tingling of hand

SPECIAL CONSIDERATION
- Fatigue rather than TOS may limit performance

REFERENCE
1. Magee DJ. *Orthopedic Physical Assessment.* 5th ed. St. Louis, MO: Saunders; 2008.

PERIPHERAL VASCULAR SYSTEM

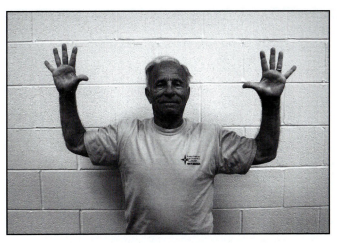

FIGURE 4-28. ROOS TEST: OPEN HANDS.

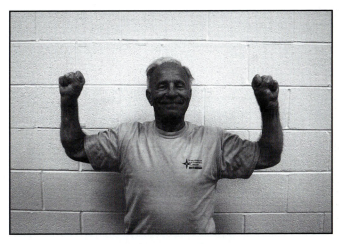

FIGURE 4-29. ROOS TEST: CLOSED HANDS.

ANKLE-BRACHIAL INDEX (ABI)

TEST POSITION
- Supine, resting for at least 5 minutes

ACTION
- Measure and record bilateral systolic pressure over the brachial artery and dorsalis pedis or tibialis anterior
- Apply conductive gel; hold Doppler probe at 50° from vertical
- Adjust probe angle and location to obtain best auditory signal
- Increase pressure in cuff ~30 mm Hg above last Korotkoff sound
- Deflate cuff pressure slowly ~2 mm Hg per second
- Record pressures and calculate ABI
- R leg/R arm pressure and L leg/R arm pressure

NORMAL FINDINGS
- 0.901 to 1.22

POSITIVE FINDINGS[1]

Table 4-5

POSITIVE ANKLE-BRACHIAL INDEX FINDINGS

Score	Diagnosis
>1.3	False positive, arterial disease, or diabetes
0.71-0.90	Mild arterial disease, perhaps claudication
0.41-0.70	Moderate arterial disease, claudication, rest pain
<0.40	Severe pain, rest pain

Adapted from Khan NA, Rahim SA, Anand SS, Simel DL, Panju A. Does the clinical examination predict lower extremity peripheral arterial disease? *JAMA*. 2006;295:536-546.

- Values <0.90 identify angiographically proven occlusions or stenoses with a sensitivity of 95% and specificity of 94% to 100%[1]

SPECIAL CONSIDERATIONS
- ABI should be assessed in individuals with
  - ◇ Diabetes who are over 50 years of age

- ✧ Diabetes who are under 50 years of age with PAD risk factors or duration of diabetes more than 10 years
- ✧ Symptoms of PAD[2]
- Postexercise ABI decrease ≥25% in claudicants is diagnostic of PAD[2]
- Low intra-observer variability (≤7.0%), high validity in detecting stenosis[3]
- 90% sensitivity, 98% specificity[3]

REFERENCES

1. Khan NA, Rahim SA, Anand SS, Simel DL, Panju A. Does the clinical examination predict lower extremity peripheral arterial disease? *JAMA.* 2006;295:536-546.

2. American Diabetes Association. Peripheral arterial disease in people with diabetes. *Diabetes Care.* 2003;26:3333-3341.

3. Doobay AV, Ananad SS. Sensitivity and specificity of the ankle brachial index to predict future cardiovascular outcomes: a systematic review. *Arteriosder Thromb Vascular Biol.* 2005;25:1463-1469.

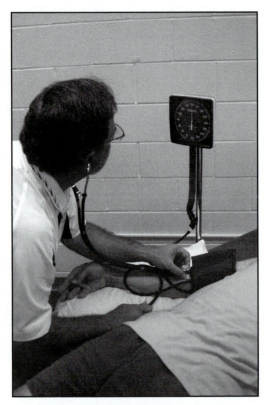

FIGURE 4-30. ABI ARM BLOOD PRESSURE
MEASUREMENT.

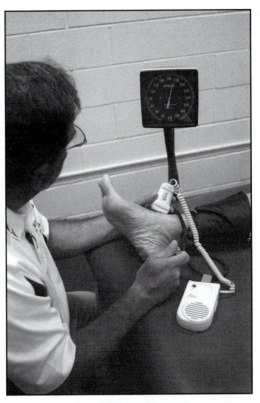

FIGURE 4-31. ABI LEG BLOOD PRESSURE
MEASUREMENT.

HOMANS' TEST

TEST POSITION
- Supine with knee flexed, hand on calf and dorsal foot

ACTION
- Forcibly and abruptly dorsiflex the client's talocrural joint and assess for pain in the posterior calf and popliteal region

NORMAL FINDINGS
- Report of stretching sensation

POSITIVE FINDINGS
- Report of pain, often excruciating upon dorsiflexion

SPECIAL CONSIDERATIONS
- Other conditions that elicit a positive Homans' sign: Calf muscle spasm or shortening, neurogenic leg pain, ruptured Baker cyst, and cellulitis
- In those with known deep vein thromboses (DVTs), accuracy of this test ranges from 8% to 56%[1]
- Homans' test has been shown to be positive in more than 50% of symptomatic patients without DVT[1]
- This test continues be used in clinical practice because of its utility and historical precedent but has poor sensitivity and specificity

REFERENCE
1. Urbano FL. Homans' sign in the diagnosis of deep venous thrombosis. *Hospital Physician.* 2001;3:22-24.

PERIPHERAL
VASCULAR SYSTEM

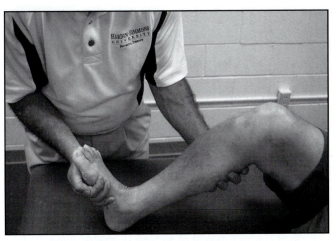

FIGURE 4-32. HOMANS' TEST.

WELLS CLINICAL PREDICTION RULE FOR DEEP VEIN THROMBOSIS

ACTION

- Obtain information from chart review, history, and/or evaluation
- Add points; note probability of DVT
- Treat or refer patient based on probability of DVT

Table 4-6
CLINICAL DECISION RULE

Clinical Finding[1]	Score[a]
Active cancer (within 6 months of diagnosis or palliative care)	1
Paralysis, paresis, or recent plaster immobilization of the lower extremity	1
Recently bedridden >3 days or major surgery within 4 weeks of application of clinical decision rule	1
Localized tenderness along the distribution of the deep venous system[b]	1
Entire lower extremity swollen	1
Calf swelling by >3 cm when compared with asymptomatic lower extremity[c]	1
Pitting edema (greater in symptomatic lower extremity)	1
Collateral superficial veins (nonvaricose)	1
Alternative diagnosis as likely or more possible than that of deep vein thrombosis[d]	-2

[a] Score interpretation: ≤ 0 = probability of proximal lower extremity deep vein thrombosis (PDVT) of 3% (95% confidence interval [CI] = 1.7%-5.9%) 1 or 2 = probability of PDVT of 17% (95% CI = 12%-23%), ≥ 3 = probability of PDVT of 75% (95% CI = 63%-84%).

[b] Tenderness along the deep venous system is assessed by firm palpation in posterior calf center, the popliteal space, and along the area of the femoral vein in the anterior thigh and groin

[c] Measured 10 cm below tibial tuberosity

[d] Most common alternative diagnoses are cellulite, calf strain, and postoperative swelling

Developed by Wells and colleagues. Reproduced with permission from Riddle DL, Wells PS. Diagnosis of lower-extremity deep vein thrombosis in outpatients. *Phys Ther.* 2004;84:729-738.

FINDINGS[1]

- A score of 1, 2, or greater indicates a probability of 3%, 17%, and 75%, respectively[1]

SPECIAL CONSIDERATIONS

- Study utilizing 110 primary care providers and 1295 consecutive patients underestimated DVTs in low-risk patients even when a D-dimer test was administered[2]
- Study of more than 1000 patients noted that DVT can be ruled out in patients with low Wells prediction scores who had negative D-dimer tests[3]

REFERENCES

1. Riddle DL, Wells PS. Diagnosis of lower-extremity deep vein thrombosis in outpatients. *Phys Ther.* 2004;84:729-738.
2. Oudega R, Hoes AW, Moons KGM. The Wells rule does not adequately rule out deep venous thrombosis in primary care patients. *Ann Intern Med.* 2005;143:100-107.
3. Wells PS, Anderson DR, Rodger M, et al. Evaluation of D-dimer in the diagnosis of suspected deep vein thrombosis. *N Engl J Med.* 2003;349:1227-1235.

WELLS CLINICAL PREDICTION RULE FOR PULMONARY EMBOLISM

ACTION

- Obtain information from chart review, history, and evaluation
- Add points for specific clinical features to determine probability of pulmonary embolism (PE)[1]

Table 4-7

VARIABLES TO DETERMINE PATIENT SCORE FOR PULMONARY EMBOLISM

Clinical Findings	Points
Clinical symptoms of DVT (minimum of leg swelling and pain with palpation of deep veins)	3.0
An alternative diagnosis is less likely than PE	3.0
Heart rate >100 beats/minute	1.5
Immobilization[a] or surgery in the previous 4 weeks	1.5
Previous DVT or PE[b]	1.5
Hemoptysis	1.0
Malignancy (on treatment, treated in the last 6 months, or palliative)	1.0

[a] ≥3 consecutive days (except for bathroom privileges)
[b] Objectively diagnosed

Reproduced with permission from Wells PS, Anderson DR, Rodger M, et al. Derivation of a simple clinical model to categorize patients probability of pulmonary embolism: increasing the models utility with the SimpliRED D-dimer. *Thromb Haemost.* 2000;83:416-420.

NORMAL FINDINGS

- Scores below 2 are least likely to predict PE

POSITIVE FINDINGS[2]

Table 4-8

SCORING FOR WELLS RULE FOR PULMONARY EMBOLISM

Score	*Probability of PE*	*Risk Status*
<2	3.4%	Low
2-6	27.8%	Moderate
≥7	78.4%	High

Adapted from Wells PS, Anderson DR, Rodger M, et al. Derivation of a simple clinical model to categorize patients probability of pulmonary embolism: increasing the models utility with the SimpliRED D-dimer. *Thromb Haemost.* 2000;83:416-420.

SPECIAL CONSIDERATIONS

- Prediction rule is easy to use but limited due to lack of a standardized method for determining whether another diagnosis is less likely than a PE
- Subjective impression remains an important component of any examination[3]

REFERENCES

1. Wells PS, Anderson DR, Rodger M, et al. Derivation of a simple clinical model to categorize patients probability of pulmonary embolism: increasing the models utility with the SimpliRED D-dimer. *Thromb Haemost.* 2000;83:416-420.

2. Wells PS, Anderson DR, Rodger M, et al. Excluding pulmonary embolism at the bedside without diagnostic imaging: management of patients with suspected pulmonary embolism presenting to the emergency department by using a simple clinical model and D-dimer. *Ann Intern Med.* 2001;135:98-107.

3. The PIOPED Investigators. Value of the ventilation/perfusion scan in acute pulmonary embolism: results of the prospective investigation of pulmonary embolism diagnosis (PIOPED). *JAMA.* 1990;263:2753-2759.

PERIPHERAL
VASCULAR SYSTEM

CLINICAL PREDICTION RULE FOR
UPPER EXTREMITY DEEP VEIN THROMBOSIS

ACTION

- Obtain information from chart review, history, evaluation
- Total 4-item scale based on specific clinical features

Table 4-9

INDEPENDENT PREDICTORS OF
UPPER EXTREMITY DEEP VEIN THROMBOSIS

Points	*Clinical Features*
+1	Venous material within the subclavian or jugular vein or a pacemaker
+1	Localized arm pain
+1	Unilateral pitting edema
-1	Alternative diagnosis at least as probable as upper extremity DVT

Reproduced with permission from Costans J, Salmi LR, Sevestre-Pietri MA, et al. A clinical prediction score for upper extremity deep venous thrombosis. *Throm Haemost.* 2008;99:202-207.

NORMAL FINDINGS

- No history of subclavian or jugular vein access, intravenous pacemaker, localized pain, or unilateral pitting edema

POSITIVE FINDINGS

- Results from 3 samples used to derive prediction rule

- Percentage of sample that had an upper extremity DVT along with 95% confidence interval

Table 4-10

SCORING FOR CLINICAL PREDICTION RULE FOR UPPER EXTREMITY DEEP VEIN THROMBOSIS

Score	Derivation Sample	Internal Validation Sample	External Validation Sample
	36/100 hospitalized patients with UEDVT	46/100 patients with UEDVT	35% of 8256 patients with UEDVT
≤0	12% (10-23)*	9% (0-20)	13% (6-19)
1	20% (9-30)	37% (19-55)	38% (27-50)
≥2	70% (57-83)	64% (51-77)	69% (54-85)

Score	External Validation Sample
	35% of 8256 patients with UEDVT
≤0	13% (6-19)*
1	38% (27-50)
≥2	69% (54-85)

*95% confidence interval

Adapted from Costans J, Salmi LR, Sevestre-Pietri MA, et al. A clinical prediction score for upper extremity deep venous thrombosis. *Throm Haemost.* 2008;99:202-207.

SPECIAL CONSIDERATION
- Excellent screening tool

REFERENCE
1. Costans J, Salmi LR, Sevestre-Pietri MA, et al. A clinical prediction score for upper extremity deep venous thrombosis. *Throm Haemost.* 2008;99:202-207.

CUFF TEST FOR VENOUS INSUFFICIENCY/OCCLUSION

TEST POSITION
- Supine

ACTION
- Place blood pressure cuff around lower leg and inflate
  - ✧ Stop upon comments of intolerable pain
  - ✧ Compare pressure readings of each leg

NORMAL FINDINGS
- Ability to withstand >40 mm Hg cuff pressure on lower leg[1]
- Equal pressure tolerance in both legs

POSITIVE FINDINGS
- Inability to withstand 40 mm Hg of cuff pressure on lower leg[1]
- Large difference in pressure tolerance between legs, with markedly lower pressure tolerance in painful or symptomatic leg (Lowenberg sign)[3]

SPECIAL CONSIDERATIONS
- Positive test results suggest a high probability of an active DVT
- This test can be augmented by a forceful squeeze of the calf region or passive dorsiflexion of the calf (Homans' sign)
- The cuff test elicits the Lowenberg sign, which has a high specificity (0.85) and low sensitivity.[3] (Some have questioned the specificity and sensitivity of this test)
- Use this test in conjunction with the Wells clinical decision-making rules for DVT

REFERENCES
1. Knight CA. Peripheral vascular disease and wound care. In: O'Sullivan SB, Schmitz TJ. *Physical Rehabilitation: Assessment and Treatment.* 4th ed. Philadelphia, PA: FA Davis Company; 2001.
2. Haeger K. Problems of acute deep venous thrombosis. I. The interpretation of signs and symptoms. *Angiology.* 1969;20:219-223.
3. Kahn SR. The clinical diagnosis of deep venous thrombosis. *Arch Int Med.* 2001;158:2315-2323.

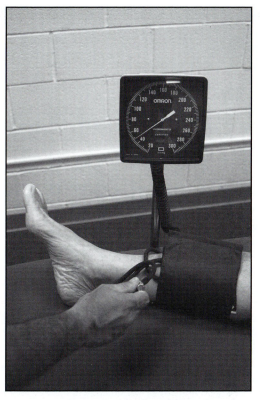

FIGURE 4-33. CUFF TEST.

VENOUS PERCUSSION, TAP, OR COUGH TEST

TEST POSITION

- Standing, weight supported on nontest leg

ACTION

- Palpate great[1] saphenous vein 6 to 8 inches distal to knee
- Tap saphenofemoral junction (SFJ)[1] or great saphenous vein proximal to knee[2] with fingertips
- Ask client to cough and palpate distal vein

NORMAL FINDINGS

- No wave of fluid is detected under distal palpation site when tapping proximal site

POSITIVE FINDINGS

- Wave of fluid detected under distal palpation site[3]

SPECIAL CONSIDERATIONS

- Fluid wave indicates incompetent valves between the SFJ and LSV at the level of the knee indicating reflux in the proximal LSV[1,3]
- Percussion test has a low sensitivity (0.18) and high specificity (0.92) and should be combined with other clinical tests or a Doppler examination[1]
- Greater or great saphenous vein starts above medial malleolus, moves anterior to medial gastrocnemius, and up through medial thigh
- Doppler can be used rather than palpation[4]

REFERENCES

1. Kim J, Richards S, Kent PJ. Clinical examination of varicose veins: a validation study. *Ann R Coll Surg Engl.* 2000;82:171-175.
2. Knight CA. Peripheral vascular disease and wound care. In: O'Sullivan SB, Schmitz TJ. *Physical Rehabilitation: Assessment and Treatment.* 4th ed. Philadelphia, PA: FA Davis Company; 2001.
3. Browse NL, Burnand KG, Irvine AT, Wilson NM, eds. *Diseases of the Veins.* 2nd ed. London: Arnold; 1998.
4. Lampe KE. Lower extremity chronic venous disease. *Cardiopulm Phys Ther.* 2004;15:13-22.

PERIPHERAL VASCULAR SYSTEM

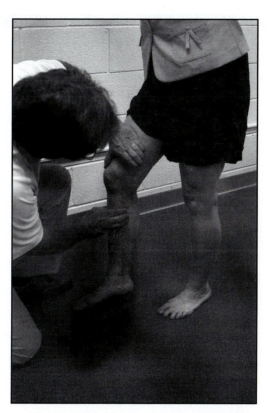

FIGURE 4-34. VENOUS PERCUSSION TEST.

VENOUS FILLING TIME

TEST POSITION
- Seated, supine, with legs dangling

ACTION
- Mark veins on dorsum of foot while in dependent position
- Supine, elevate legs to 45° for 1 minute
- Rapidly change position to sitting, dangling legs/feet
- Observe and record when veins bulge above skin surface

FINDINGS

Table 4-11

VENOUS FILLING TIMES

Vascular Component	Normal Refill	Time for Refill	Positive Findings
Arterial	~15-20 sec Pink color	>20 seconds[1]	Suggests arterial insufficiency[1]
Venous	>30 sec[2-4]	<30 seconds[1]	Suggests venous incompetence[2-4]

SPECIAL CONSIDERATIONS
- Specificity: 94%, sensitivity: 22% in diabetic sample[3]
- Very rapid venous filling suggests venous disease
- Very slowly returning pink coloration suggests arterial disease

REFERENCES
1. Lampe KE. Lower extremity chronic venous disease. *Cardiopulm Phys Ther.* 2004;15:13-22.
2. Boyko EJ, Ahroni JH, Davignon D, Stensel V, Prigeon RL, Smith DG. Diagnostic utility of the history and physical examination for peripheral vascular disease among patients with diabetes mellitus. *J Clin Epidemiol.* 1997;50:659-668.

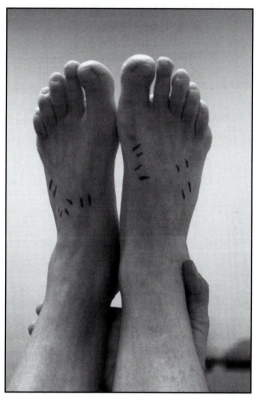

FIGURE 4-35. ELEVATED LEGS.

PERIPHERAL
VASCULAR SYSTEM

3. Kozak GP, Hoar CS, Rowbotham JL, Wheelock FC, Gibbons GW, Campbell D, eds. *Management of Diabetic Feet Problems*. Philadelphia, PA: WB Saunders; 1994.

4. Sammarco GJ, Scvioli MW. Examination of the foot and ankle. In: Sammarco GJ, ed. *The Foot in Diabetes*. Philadelphia, PA: Lea and Febiger; 1991:33.

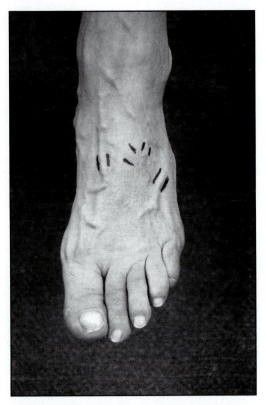

FIGURE 4-36. DANGLING, MARKED, FILLED VEINS.

PITTING EDEMA

TEST POSITION

- Feet or other body part (eg, hand) in a dependent position

ACTION

- Apply digital pressure for 15 to 30 seconds over bony prominence[1]

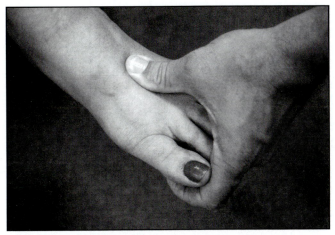

FIGURE 4-37. PRESSURE APPLIED TO FOOT.

- Determine soft (pitting) vs indurated (nonpitting edema)

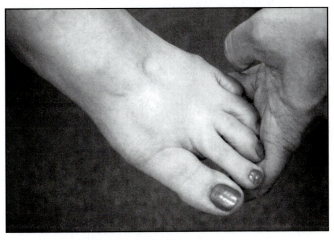

FIGURE 4-38. PITTING EDEMA.

- Grade edema based on depth or record time required for tissue normalization

POSITIVE FINDINGS

- Edema resolving in <4 seconds suggests hypoalbuminemia[2]
- Edema resolving in >40 seconds suggests congestive heart failure[2]

Table 4-12

PITTING EDEMA GRADES (DEPTH)[1] OR APPEARANCE[3]

Depth[1]

Depth (mm)	5	10	15	20	25	30	>35
Grade	1/7	2/7	3/7	4/7	5/7	6/7	7/7

Appearance[3]

1+ Mild pitting, slight indentation, no leg swelling

2+ Moderate pitting, rapid loss of indentation

3+ Deep pitting, indentation remains for short period, swollen leg

4+ Very deep pitting with long-lasting indentation, very swollen leg

Adapted from Nelson JP. The vascular history and physical examination. *Clin Pod Med Surg.* 1992;9:1-13 and Jarvis C. *Physical Examination and Health Assessment.* 5th ed. St. Louis, MO: Saunders-Elsevier; 2008.

SPECIAL CONSIDERATIONS

- Common causes of pitting edema are systemic origin, local origin, drug induced, or other causes
- Edema may have venous, arteriolar, capillary, extravascular compartments, or lymphatic causes[2]
- Time to pit resolution can be used rather than depth
- Differences between lymphedema and edema (Table 4-13)

REFERENCES

1. Nelson JP. The vascular history and physical examination. *Clin Pod Med Surg.* 1992;9:1-13.
2. Yale SH, Mazza JJ. Approach to diagnosing lower extremity edema. *Compr Ther.* 2001;27:242-252.
3. Jarvis C. *Physical Examination and Health Assessment.* 5th ed. St. Louis, MO: Saunders-Elsevier; 2008.

Table 4-13

LYMPHEDEMA VS VENOUS STASIS EDEMA

Features of Edema	Lymphedema	Venous Stasis
Onset	Varies	Often with aging
Location	70% unilateral	Uni- or bilateral
Skin	Thick, hyperkeratotic, dermal fibrosis in late stages	Weeping, erosions, excoriation
Tissue consistency	Doughy, may be hard in later stages	Very soft
Tenderness	Minimal	None
Ulcers	No	Yes, frequently at medial malleolus
Effect of elevation	Minimal early, rare effect late in disease	Beneficial
Coloration		Brown

Adapted from Yale SH, Mazza JJ. Approach to diagnosing lower extremity edema. *Compr Ther.* 2001;27:242-252.

KAPOSI STEMMER SIGN (EDEMA VS LYMPHEDEMA)

TEST POSITION
- Supine

ACTION
- Pick up a skinfold over the dorsum of the second toe[1]

NORMAL FINDINGS
- A skinfold can be pinched[1]

POSITIVE FINDINGS
- A skinfold that cannot be pinched[1] suggests lymphedema

SPECIAL CONSIDERATIONS
- A skinfold may be pinched on an edematous limb but not on a limb with chronic lymphedema[1]
- Early lymphedema and venous edema may be indistinguishable with this test[1]
- Acutely occurring (<72 hours) unilateral edema, likely DVT[1]
- Chronic unilateral edema, likely chronic venous insufficiency[1]
- Chronic bilateral edema may be due to venous, cardiac, arteriolar/capillary, pulmonary, and lymphatic causations or may be due to hypoalbuminemia, premenstruation, medications, obesity, pregnancy[1,2]
- Clients with lymphedema and/or venous stasis edema can have cellulitis, foot involvement, and pitting

REFERENCES
1. Ely JW, Osheroff JA, Chambliss ML, Ebell MH. Approach to leg edema of unclear etiology. *J Am Board Fam Med.* 2006;19:148-160.
2. Yale SH, Mazza JJ. Approach to diagnosing lower extremity edema. *Compr Ther.* 2001;27:242-252.

PERIPHERAL VASCULAR SYSTEM

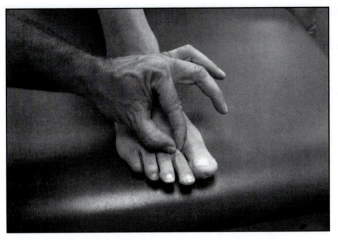

FIGURE 4-39. PINCHING SKIN OVER SECOND TOE.

AUSCULTATION OF CAROTID ARTERY

TEST POSITION
- Seated or supine, head turned slightly away from examiner[1]

ACTION
- Place stethoscope bell at angle of jaw, carotid bifurcation, base of neck, then subclavian arteries
- Client inhales, exhales, and holds breath for 15 seconds[1]
- Auscultation occurs during and immediately following exhalation
- Examiner listens for continuous murmurs[1] (systolic-diastolic)

NORMAL FINDINGS
- Sometimes a pulse is heard
- Cervical venous hums are normal in children and young adults[1]
- Venous hums disappear or decrease in supine

POSITIVE FINDINGS
- A carotid, systolic bruit is a blowing, swishing sound suggesting turbulence
- Carotid bruits augmented or unchanged in recumbency[1]

SPECIAL CONSIDERATIONS
- A pulse is normally heard but without sounds during systole
- Innocent supraclavicular systolic bruits are often heard in normal children or adolescents
- Carotid bruits are rare in children and young adults[1]
- Carotid bruits are powerful screening tests for internal carotid artery stenosis[2,3]
- Subclavian artery sounds are obliterated with shoulder extension
- Excess pressure over the carotids can mimic a murmur[1]
- Venous hum is a murmur best heard just above the right clavicle and may radiate into the neck
- Carotid bruits have a high specificity (>90%) for detection of carotid artery stenosis and is a useful indicator of systemic atherosclerosis[4]

PERIPHERAL
VASCULAR SYSTEM

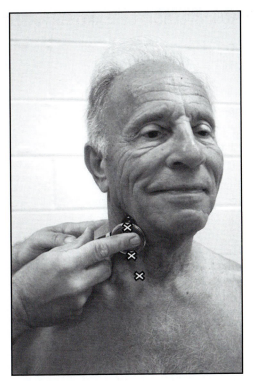

FIGURE 4-40. CAROTID AUSCULTATION.

REFERENCES

1. Wilms JL, Schneiderman H. *Physical Diagnosis.* Baltimore, MD: Williams & Wilkins; 1996.

2. Jarvis C. *Physical Examination and Health Assessment.* 5th ed. St. Louis, MO: Saunders-Elsevier; 2008.

3. Richardson DA, Shaw FE, Bexton R, Steen N, Kenny RA. Presence of a carotid bruit in adults with unexplained or recurrent falls: implications for carotid sinus massage. *Age Ageing.* 2002;31:379-384.

4. Paraskevas KI, Hamilton G, Mikhailidis DP. Clinical significance of carotid bruits: an innocent finding or a useful warning sign? *Neurol Res.* 2008;30:523-530.

Section

FIVE

Submaximal
Exercise Evaluation

CONCEPTS OF SUBMAXIMAL TESTING

PURPOSE
- To predict maximal oxygen consumption (VO_2max) and to determine if exercise responses at submaximal levels progress normally

SPECIFICITY
- Testing should be specific to the client's work, sport, or avocation
- Test runners on treadmills, cyclists on cycle ergometers, sailors on arm crank ergometers
- Use other ergometers if they can be calibrated

STEADY-STATE METABOLISM
- Steady-state occurs at a constant workload after 2 to 3 minutes
- Steady-state VO_2 occurs below the anaerobic threshold
- Heart rate, an indirect measure of metabolism, should increase with increasing work but not vary less than ±5 beats/minute during the 2nd and 3rd minute of a low-intensity workload

NONSTEADY-STATE METABOLISM
- Metabolism becomes increasingly anaerobic as intensity increases
  - ✧ In the unfit, this can be as low as 65% of VO_2max
  - ✧ In the highly fit, this may be very close to 100% of VO_2max

BENEFITS OF SUBMAXIMAL TESTING
- Heart rate, blood pressure, rating of perceived exertion, SpO_2, and other physiological and perceptual parameters can be used in educating the client in a real-time exercise experience
- Abnormalities can be noted at specific intensities and then exercise can be prescribed at an intensity 10 to 15 beats/minute below any unusual findings[1]

REFERENCES
1. American College of Sports Medicine. *ACSM Guidelines for Exercise Testing and Prescription.* 7th ed. Philadelphia, PA: Lippincott Williams & Wilkins; 2006.

O'Connell DG, O'Connell JK, Hinman MR.
Special Tests of the Cardiopulmonary, Vascular and Gastrointestinal Systems (pp 198-262).
© 2011 SLACK Incorporated

OXYGEN CONSUMPTION AND METs

GENERAL CONCEPTS

- Maximal oxygen uptake (VO_2max) is the criterion measure of cardiorespiratory fitness
  - ✧ The maximal amount of oxygen consumed during exercise
- Oxygen consumption is measured at rest through maximal exertion
- Expired air is measured for volume and expired O_2 and CO_2 content
- Clients progress through several submaximal levels of exercise until they can no longer continue

CRITERIA FOR ACHIEVING MAXIMUM OXYGEN CONSUMPTION[1]

- VO_2 fails to increase by 150 mL·min^{-1} with increasing workload
- Heart rate fails to increase with increasing workload[1]
- Respiratory exchange ratio >1.1
- Rate of perceived exertion reaches >17/20 or 10/10
- Postexercise venous blood lactate level >8 mmol
- Maximal oxygen consumption, maximal aerobic capacity, maximal aerobic power, or uptake are synonymous

EXPRESSIONS OF OXYGEN CONSUMPTION

- Maximal or submaximal VO_2 values are typically expressed as mL·kg^{-1}·min^{-1} which is considered relative to body weight
- Relative $VO_2 \div 3.5$ = metabolic equivalent
- 1 metabolic equivalent = 1 MET
- 1 MET = 3.5 mL·kg^{-1}·min^{-1}
- Oxygen consumption can be expressed in absolute terms (liters/minute)

CONVERSION FACTORS

- 1 MET = 3.5 mL·kg^{-1}·min^{-1}
- Clients consume 3.5 mL of O_2/ minute^{-1} for every kg (2.2 lbs)
- 1 L = 1000 mL
- 1 L of oxygen consumed = 5.0 kcals of heat energy

REFERENCE

1. American College of Sports Medicine. *ACSM Guidelines for Exercise Testing and Prescription.* 7th ed. Philadelphia, PA: Lippincott Williams & Wilkins; 2006.

SUBMAXIMAL EXERCISE

METABOLIC EQUIVALENTS (METs)

GENERAL CONCEPTS
- METs are shorthand for oxygen consumption
- 1 MET = 3.5 mL·kg^{-1}·min^{-1}
- 1 MET = supine or seated rest
- All rest or work tasks represent a percentage of max METs
- Eating requires a metabolic rate slightly higher than rest
- The intensity of an activity relates to max METs
- Work task METs= [max METs -1 (rest) x intensity] + rest METs

Table 5-1
ADL WORK TASKS AND MET LEVELS[1]

Task	METs[1]	Relative % of 5 MET Max
Rest	1	20
Eating or playing cards	1.4	35
Baking	2.1	53
Food shopping or mopping floor	3.5	88
Cleaning or dusting	3.6	90
Laundry	3.7	93
Window washing	3.8	96
Garden digging	4.1	103
Car wash	4.2	105
Vacuuming	5.0	125

Adapted from McArdle WD, Katch FI, Katch VL. *Exercise Physiology: Energy, Nutrition, and Human Performance.* 6th ed. Philadelphia, PA: Lippincott Williams & Wilkins; 2007.

- Exercise capacity <5 METs indicates an increased risk for mortality[2]
- Encourage all children and adults to train their cardiopulmonary systems to increase their max MET level as high as possible

SUBMAXIMAL EXERCISE

- The higher the max MET level, the less intense any given work task
- MET tables are likely based on small sample sizes and likely have inherent errors[3]

REFERENCES

1. McArdle WD, Katch FI, Katch VL. *Exercise Physiology: Energy, Nutrition, and Human Performance.* 6th ed. Philadelphia, PA: Lippincott Williams & Wilkins; 2007.
2. Franklin BA. Survival of the fittest: evidence for high-risk and cardioprotective fitness levels. *Curr Sports Med Rep.* 2002;5:257-259.
3. O'Connell DG, O'Connell JK. A MET isn't just a baseball player from New York. *WORK.* 1994;4:220-222.

MEASURING EXERCISE HEART RATE

TESTING CONDITION
- Exercise: Subject seated, semirecumbent, supine, standing

ACTION
- May be measured for 10, 15, 30, or 60 sec

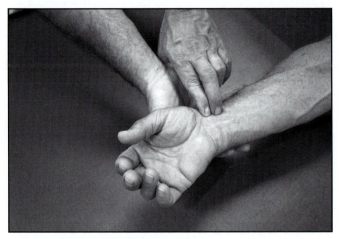

FIGURE 5-1. MEASUREMENT OF RADIAL PULSE.

- 10 to 15 sec is most practical
- Heart rates for the last portion (10 to 15 sec) of the final 2 minutes of most workloads are averaged
- Exercise heart rate via palpation or auscultation
  See Table 5-2 on the following page.
- Exercise heart rate via chest strap receiver
  ✧ Average heart rates for last 5 to 10 seconds of each workload

NORMAL FINDINGS
- Exercise heart rate increases with increasing intensity
- Resting heart rate may be elevated with anxious clients, decrease in early exercise, then increase
- Exercise heart rate tends to drift upward over time

Table 5-2

WHEN AND WHERE TO OBTAIN EXERCISE HEART RATES

Ergometer	Location	Time of Measurement
Arm cycle or rowing ergometer	Radial pulse or apical impulse	Immediate postworkload (10 seconds)
Leg cycle	Radial pulse or apical impulse	During exercise
Stepping	Radial pulse or apical impulse	During or immediately post-workload (10 seconds)
Treadmill	Radial pulse or apical impulse	During or immediately post-workload (10 seconds)

PREDICTING VO$_2$MAX FROM SUBMAXIMAL HEART RATE DATA

THE HR-VO$_2$ RELATIONSHIP

- Oxygen consumption and heart rate are linearly related between 110 and 150 beats/minute
- This relationship allows prediction of VO$_2$max from submaximal heart rate data
- Beta blockers, calcium channel blockers, nicotine, alcohol, and fatigue may affect this relationship

STANDARDIZED PROCEDURES

- Avoid a) strenuous activity 24 hrs pretest, b) heavy meal, caffeine, and nicotine within 2 to 3 hrs prior to testing
- Provide a practice test[1]
- Standardize verbal encouragement
- Measure as many responses as possible as often as possible (eg, HR, BP)

ACTION

- Draw horizontal line representing client's predicted HRmax[2,3]
- Subtract client's age from 220
  - ✧ Example: 30-year-old subject, nonsmoker, nonmedicated
  - ✧ Resting heart rate = 60 beats/min
  - ✧ 220 – 30 = 190 = predicted maximal heart rate
- Obtain and average heart rates for minutes 2 and 3 of each workload[2]
  - ✧ If minutes 2 and 3 heart rates differ more than 5 beats, add 1 minute and average minutes 3 and 4
- Plot steady-state heart rates for each workload[2,3]
  - ✧ Example: Steady-state heart rates of 110 and 125 at 300 and 450 kg·m·min^{-1}, respectively
  - ✧ Draw a line through exercise heart rates
  - ✧ Draw vertical line downward where the plotted heart rate line and predicted maximal heart rate line intersect (2.1 L/min^{-1})

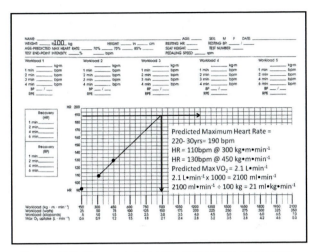

FIGURE 5-2. PLOTTING EXERCISE HEART RATES TO PREDICT
VO₂MAX. (USED WITH PERMISSION FROM GOLDING LA, ED.
YMCA FITNESS TESTING AND ASSESSMENT MANUAL, 4TH ED.
CHAMPAIGN, IL: YMCA OF THE USA; 2000.)

SPECIAL CONSIDERATIONS[1,2]

- Predicting maximal heart rate may vary ±10 to 12 beats/min[1]
- Prediction error exists when predicting VO_2max^{-1} from submaximal heart rate data

REFERENCES

1. Tonino RP, Driscoll PA. Reliability of maximal and submaximal parameters of treadmill testing for the measurement of physical training in older persons. *J Gerontol.* 1988;43:101-104.

2. American College of Sports Medicine. *ACSM Guidelines for Exercise Testing and Prescription.* 7th ed. Philadelphia, PA: Lippincott Williams & Wilkins; 2006.

3. Altug Z, Hoffman JL, Martin JL. *Manual of Clinical Exercise Testing, Prescription, and Rehabilitation.* Norwalk, CT: Appleton-Lange; 1993.

SUBMAXIMAL
EXERCISE

MAX METs NORMATIVE DATA

ACTION

- Predict or measure VO$_2$max, divide by 3.5
- Compare with normative data below

NORMAL FINDINGS

- Average or above average fitness

POSITIVE FINDINGS

- Below average fitness

Table 5-3

MAX MET NORMS

Men

Age	Poor	Fair	Average	Good	Excellent
< 29	≤ 6.9	7.1-9.7	9.7-12.5	12.6-15.1	≥ 15.1
30-39	≤ 6.5	7.1-8.8	8.9-12.0	12.1-14.3	≥ 14.3
40-49	≤ 5.7	5.7-7.7	7.7-10.8	11.1-12.8	≥ 12.8
50-59	≤ 5.1	5.1-7.1	7.1-10.8	10.9-12.3	≥ 12.3
60-69	≤ 4.5	4.6-6.5	6.6-10.3	10.3-11.7	≥ 11.7

Women

Age	Poor	Fair	Average	Good	Excellent
< 29	≤ 6.8	6.9-8.8	8.9-11.1	11.1-14.0	≥ 14.1
30-39	≤ 5.7	5.7-8.0	8.0-10.5	10.6-12.8	≥ 13.1
40-49	≤ 4.8	4.8-7.1	7.1-10.5	7.7-12.0	≥ 12.2
50-59	≤ 4.3	4.3-6.3	6.3-9.7	9.7-11.4	≥ 10.7
60-69	≤ 3.7	3.7-6.0	6.0-9.4	9.4-10.5	≥ 9.9

Adapted from McArdle WD, Katch FI, Katch VL. *Exercise Physiology: Energy, Nutrition, and Human Performance.* 6th ed. Philadelphia, PA: Lippincott Williams & Wilkins; 2007.

SUBMAXIMAL EXERCISE

RISK STRATIFICATION FOR
EXERCISE TESTING OR PRESCRIPTION

Prior to exercise testing or before initiating an aerobic exercise program, the risk of an untoward exercise event should be considered.

ACTION

- Step 1: Determine age and add number of risk factors in Table 5-4

Table 5-4

RISK FACTORS FOR CORONARY ARTERY DISEASE

Risk Factor	Defining Criteria	Further Criteria
Family Hx	Myocardial infarction, coronary artery bypass graft, stent, sudden death	Father or other 1st-degree ♂ relative prior to 55 years of age, or mother/other 1st-degree ♀ relative prior to 65 years of age
Cigarette smoking	Current or quit within past 6 months	
Hypertension	≥140 mm Hg systolic ≥90 mm Hg diastolic or takes antihypertensive medicine	2 separate occasions
Dyslipidemia	LDL ≥130 mg/dL^{-1} or HDL <40 mg/dL^{-1} or on lipid-lowering medication	If only total cholesterol is available, >200 mg/dL
Impaired fasting glucose	≥100 mg/dL^{-1}	2 separate occasions
Obesity	BMI >30 kg/m^2	Waist circumference >102 cm ♂ or >88 cm ♀
Sedentary Lifestyle	<30 minutes of moderate activity most days of the week	
High HDL	≥60 mg/dL^{-1}	Subtract from other risk factors

Adapted from American College of Sports Medicine. *ACSM Guidelines for Exercise Testing and Prescription.* 7th ed. Philadelphia, PA: Lippincott Williams & Wilkins; 2006.

- Step 2: Determine risk of an acute cardiovascular event during exercise with Table 5-5

Table 5-5

ADD RISK FACTORS AND DETERMINE RISK STATUS

Risk	Age/Gender	Risk Factors
Low	<45 yrs	0 or 1
	<55 yrs	0 or 1
Moderate	≥45 yrs	≥2
	≥55 yrs	≥2
High	Anyone with systemic disease	Cardiovascular, pulmonary, thyroid, renal, or liver disease, or diabetes

Adapted from American College of Sports Medicine. *ACSM Guidelines for Exercise Testing and Prescription.* 7th ed. Philadelphia, PA: Lippincott Williams & Wilkins; 2006.

SUBMAXIMAL EXERCISE

- Step 3: Based on the risk of an acute cardiovascular event, determine the type of supervision needed for exercise testing or an exercise program

Table 5-6

RECOMMENDATIONS FOR
FURTHER EXAMINATION AND TESTING

	Low Risk	Moderate Risk	High Risk
Further medical examination prior to exercise training	No	Yes	Yes
Further exercise testing prior to moderate[1] exercise training	No		Yes
Exercise testing needed prior to vigorous[2] exercise training		Yes	Yes
Medical supervision[3] during submaximal exercise testing	No		Yes
Medical supervision[3] during maximal exercise testing	No	Yes	Yes

[1] Moderate intensity = 40%-59% of VO_2 reserve
[2] Vigorous intensity >60% of VO_2 reserve
[3] Supervision = Doctor in close proximity to the test

Adapted from American College of Sports Medicine. *ACSM Guidelines for Exercise Testing and Prescription.* 7th ed. Philadelphia, PA: Lippincott Williams & Wilkins; 2006.

SUBMAXIMAL EXERCISE

GENERAL EXERCISE TEST PROCEDURAL INFORMATION

Prior to exercise testing or before initiating an aerobic exercise program, the risk of untoward exercise events should be considered.

BACKGROUND

- Many aerobic tests predict VO_2max and test reliability and validity should be considered
- For submaximal tests, avoid exceeding 85% of predicted maximal heart rate because typical adults planning to improve fitness need not surpass this intensity
- Calculate training heart rates prior to testing and use this information for educating the client during the test
- Calibrate equipment prior to testing
- Step tests are performed at specific step heights and stepping frequencies
- Fitness determined by most step tests requires measurement of recovery heart rate
- Mechanically braked cycle ergometer tests are performed using a calibrated cycle ergometer at a very specific pedaling frequency
- Calibrate cycle ergometers prior to the first test on each test day
- Most cycle ergometer tests require that the subject's exercise heart rate reach a particular minimal value
- Stepping and cycling frequencies can be maintained with a metronome
- Calibrate metronomes by measuring frequencies for 1 minute prior to testing
- VO_2max can be predicted utilizing several consecutive 3-minute stages of large muscle group exercise as long as the average heart rate for minutes 2 and 3 exceeds 110 beats/minute[1]
- Measure blood pressure during the last minute of an exercise stage
- Perceived exertion data and exercise heart rate information allows for client education during the exercise test
- Testing and training modalities should be identical

REFERENCE

1. American College of Sports Medicine. *ACSM Guidelines for Exercise Testing and Prescription.* 7th ed. Philadelphia, PA: Lippincott Williams & Wilkins; 2006.

SUBMAXIMAL EXERCISE

BRUCE TREADMILL PROTOCOL

ACTION

- Prepare client and calculate predicted max heart rate
- Obtain standing pretest resting physiological data (HR, BP)
- Obtain heart rate or ECG data each minute and blood pressure data in the last minute of each 3-minute exercise stage
- Client rates perceived exertion, angina, dyspnea, and claudication the last minute of each stage, or as needed
- Holding handrails or leaning on front or side handrails during testing is discouraged; if unstable, both hands may rest on, but not grip the rails

---

Table 5-7

BRUCE TREADMILL PROTOCOL (NOT HOLDING HANDRAIL)

Stage	Minute	MPH	Percent Grade	METs
1	1-3	1.7	10	4.9
2	4-6	2.5	12	7.0
3	7-9	3.4	14	10.0
4	10-12	4.2	16	13.1
5	13-15	5.0	18	16.1
6	16-18	5.5	20	19.4

Adapted from Fardy PS, Bennett JL, Reitz NL, Williams MA. *Cardiac Rehabilitation: Implications for the Nurse and Other Health Professionals.* St. Louis, MO: CV Mosby Company; 1980.

SUBMAXIMAL
EXERCISE

Table 5-8

BRUCE TREADMILL PROTOCOL
(HOLDING HANDRAIL)

Minute	MPH	Percent Grade	VO_2 $(mL \cdot kg^{-1} \cdot min^{-1})$	METs
1	1.7	10	10.8	3.1
2	1.7	10	13.1	3.7
3	1.7	10	15.4	4.4
4	2.5	12	17.7	5.0
5	2.5	12	20.0	5.7
6	2.5	12	22.2	6.4
7	3.4	14	24.5	7.0
8	3.4	14	26.8	7.7
9	3.4	14	29.1	8.3
10	4.2	16	31.4	9.0
11	4.2	16	33.7	9.6
12	4.2	16	35.9	10.3

Adapted from McConnell TR, Clark BA. Prediction of maximal oxygen consumption during handrail-supported treadmill exercise. *J Cardiopulm Rehabil.* 1987;7:324-331.

- Active cool down at self-selected walking speed (~1.5 to 2.5 mph) encouraged
- Watch for pallor and/or blood pooling in unfit and those who reach maximal exertion
- Measure blood pressure at minutes 1, 3, and 5 of recovery or as needed
- Predict VO_2max from equations (Table 5-9) if client achieves achieves near maximal heart rate
- Average heart rates from the last 2 minutes of several submaximal workloads can be used for plotting and prediction of VO_2max (see Appendix D on page 270)

Table 5-9

EQUATIONS FOR PREDICTING VO$_2$MAX FROM BRUCE TREADMILL (WITH AND WITHOUT HOLDING HANDRAILS)[1,2]

Protocol	Equation
Bruce Treadmill (without hand-rail support)	VO$_2$max (mL•kg^{-1}•min^{-1}) = 14.8 − 1.379 (time in min) + 0.451 (time^2) − 0.012 (time^3) SEE = 3.35 mL•kg^{-1}•min^{-1}
Bruce Treadmill (with handrail support)	VO$_2$max (mL•kg^{-1}•min^{-1}) = 2.282 (time in min) + 8.545 SEE = 4.92 mL•kg^{-1}•min^{-1}

SEE = standard error of the estimate

NORMAL FINDINGS

- Average and above aerobic fitness (see Appendix A on page 264)
- Increased heart rate, SBP with increasing workloads

ABNORMAL FINDINGS

- Below average fitness (see Appendix A on page 264))
- Heart rate or SBP fail to increase with increasing workloads
- Diastolic blood pressure changing ≥10 mm Hg from standing resting levels

SPECIAL CONSIDERATIONS

- Initial workload (>3 METs) and steep inclination changes may be challenging for many clients
- Static gastrocnemius and soleus muscle stretching should be encouraged before and following the test
- An active cool down is recommended to prevent blood pooling

REFERENCES

1. American College of Sports Medicine. *ACSM Guidelines for Exercise Testing and Prescription.* 7th ed. Philadelphia, PA: Lippincott Williams & Wilkins; 2006.

SUBMAXIMAL EXERCISE

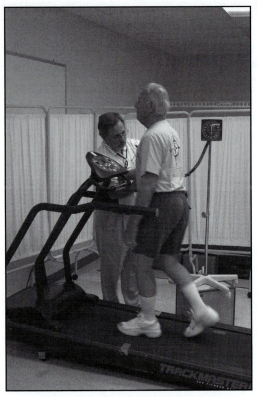

FIGURE 5-3. EXERCISE TREADMILL TEST.

2. Bruce RA, Kusumi F, Hosmer D. Maximal oxygen intake and nomographic assessment of functional aerobic impairment in cardiovascular disease. *Am Heart J.* 1973;85:546-562.

EXERCISE TEST OR EXERCISE SESSION TERMINATION

ACTION

- Participation in exercise/therapy session or in a nondiagnostic exercise test

NORMAL FINDINGS

- Heart rate, SBP, rate of perceived exertion increase with increasing workloads, and return to pre-exercise levels during recovery

POSITIVE FINDINGS

See Table 5-10 on the following pages.

SPECIAL CONSIDERATION

- Exercise is inherently safe at low intensity and in noncompetitive situations

Table 5-10

REASONS TO TERMINATE EXERCISE SESSIONS OR EXERCISE TESTS

	Reasons to Stop Non-diagnostic Fitness Test or Exercise Session Without Physician Present	Relative Reasons to Stop a Diagnostic Test or Exercise Session	Absolute Reasons to Stop a Diagnostic Test or Exercise Session
Angina	Onset of angina or angina-like symptoms	Angina rating of 1 or 2 on 4-point scale	Angina rating of 3 on a 4-point scale
Client Request	Asks to stop	Asks to stop	Asks to stop
Appearance	Appears severely fatigued	Appears severely fatigued	Unsteady gait, dizziness, loss of balance, or near fainting
Signs of Intolerance	Shortness of breath, wheezing, leg cramps, claudication	Shortness of breath, wheezing, leg cramps, claudication plus fatigue	Shortness of breath, wheezing, leg cramps, claudication plus fatigue
Signs of Poor Perfusion	Light-headedness, confusion, ataxia, pallor, cyanosis, nausea, or cold, clammy skin		Light-headedness, confusion, ataxia, pallor, cyanosis, nausea, or cold, clammy skin

(continued)

Table 5-10 (continued)

REASONS TO TERMINATE EXERCISE SESSIONS OR EXERCISE TESTS

	Reasons to Stop Non-diagnostic Fitness Test or Exercise Session Without Physician Present	Relative Reasons to Stop a Diagnostic Test or Exercise Session	Absolute Reasons to Stop a Diagnostic Test or Exercise Session
SBP Decrease	SBP drops >10 mm Hg from baseline with increase in workload	SBP drops >10 mm Hg from baseline with increase in workload without evidence of ischemia	SBP drops >10 mm Hg from baseline with increase in workload with evidence of ischemia
BP Elevation	SBP and DBP rise to >250 and >115 mm Hg	SBP and DBP rise to >250 and >115 mm Hg	SBP and DBP rise to >250 and >115 mm Hg
Equipment Malfunction	Any malfunction	Any malfunction	ECG, BP equipment failure
Heart Rate	Fails to increase as workloads increase		

(continued)

SUBMAXIMAL
EXERCISE

Table 5-10 (continued)

REASONS TO TERMINATE EXERCISE SESSIONS OR EXERCISE TESTS

	Reasons to Stop Non-diagnostic Fitness Test or Exercise Session Without Physician Present	Relative Reasons to Stop a Diagnostic Test or Exercise Session	Absolute Reasons to Stop a Diagnostic Test or Exercise Session
Arrhythmias	Palpable/auscultatory rhythm changes from rest	Multifocal PVCs, PVC-triplets, supraventricular tachycardia, heart block, bradyarrhythmia, bundle, branch block, or conduction delay similar to ventricular tachycardia	Sustained ventricular tachycardia or worsening multifocal PVCs, PVC-triplets, supraventricular tachycardia, heart block, bradyarrhythmia, bundle, branch block, or conduction delay
ST Elevation			ST elevation (≥ 1 mm) in leads without diagnostic Q-waves other than V1 or AVR
ST Segment Depression		Horizontal or downsloping ST depression > 2 mm	Horizontal or downsloping ST depression > 2 mm
QRS Changes		Marked axis shift	Marked axis shift

Adapted from American College of Sports Medicine. ACSM Guidelines for Exercise Testing and Prescription. 7th ed. Philadelphia, PA: Lippincott Williams & Wilkins; 2006.

PREDICTION OF VO$_2$MAX VIA NONEXERCISE SURVEY

ACTION

- Measure height and weight and compute BMI
- Complete Perceived Functional Ability Questions

Table 5-11

PERCEIVED FUNCTIONAL ABILITY QUESTIONS

1. Suppose you were going to exercise on an indoor track for 1 mile. Which exercise pace is just right for you—not too easy and not too hard? Circle the number that most accurately describes your current ability (any number, 1 to 13).

   1   Walking at a slow pace (18 min per mile or more)

   2

   3   Walking at a medium pace (16 min per mile)

   4

   5   Walking at a fast pace (14 min per mile)

   6

   7   Jogging at a slow pace (12 min per mile)

   8

   9   Jogging at a medium pace (10 min per mile)

   10

   11   Jogging at a fast pace (8 min per mile)

   12

   13   Running at a fast, competitive pace (7 min per mile or less)

   (continued)

SUBMAXIMAL
EXERCISE

Table 5-11 (continued)

PERCEIVED FUNCTIONAL ABILITY QUESTIONS

2. How fast could you cover a distance of 3 miles and NOT become breathless or overly fatigued? Be realistic.
    Circle the number that most accurately describes your current ability (any number, 1 to 13).

1	I could walk the entire distance at a slow pace (18 min per mile or more)
2	
3	I could walk the entire distance at a medium pace (16 min per mile)
4	
5	I could walk the entire distance at a fast pace (14 min per mile)
6	
7	I could jog the entire distance at a slow pace (12 min per mile)
8	
9	I could jog the entire distance at a medium pace (10 min per mile)
10	
11	I could jog the entire distance at a fast pace (8 min per mile)
12	
13	I could run the entire distance at a fast, competitive pace (7 min per mile or less)

Modified from George JD, Stone WJ, Burkett LN. Non-exercise VO₂max estimation for physically active college students. *Med Sci Sports Exerc.* 1997;29(3):415-423.

- Complete Physical Activity Rating Questions
  See Table 5-12 on the following page.
- Calculate predicted VO_2max[1] and compare to normative data
  VO_2max $(mL \cdot kg^{-1} \cdot min^{-1})$ = 48.073 + 6.1779 (gender: ♀ = 0, ♂ = 1) − 0.2463 (age) − 0.6186 (BMI) + 0.715 (PFA) + 0.679 (PA-R)

NORMAL FINDINGS

- Average to excellent predicted VO_2max values

Table 5-12

PHYSICAL ACTIVITY RATING (PA-R) QUESTIONS

Select the number that best describes your overall level of physical activity for the previous 6 months:

0 = Avoid walking or exertion: always use elevator, drive when possible instead of walking

1 = Light activity: walk for pleasure, routinely use stairs, occasionally exercise sufficiently to cause heavy breathing or perspiration

2 = Moderate activity: 10 to 60 minutes per week of moderate activity such as golf, horseback riding, calisthenics, table tennis, bowling, weightlifting, yard work, cleaning house, walking for exercise

3 = Moderate activity: more than 1 hour per week of moderate activity as described above

4 = Vigorous activity: run less than 1 mile per week or spend less than 30 minutes per week in comparable activity such as running or jogging, lap swimming, cycling, rowing, aerobics, skipping rope, running in place, or engaging in vigorous aerobic-type activity such as soccer, basketball, tennis, racquetball, or handball

5 = Vigorous activity: run 1 mile to less than 5 miles per week or spend 30 minutes to less than 60 minutes per week in comparable physical activity as described above

6 = Vigorous activity: run 5 miles to less than 10 miles per week or spend 1 hour to less than 3 hours per week in comparable physical activity as described above

7 = Vigorous activity: run 10 miles to less than 15 miles per week or spend 3 hours to less than 6 hours per week in comparable physical activity as described above

8 = Vigorous activity: run 15 miles to less than 20 miles per week or spend 6 hours to less than 7 hours per week in comparable physical activity as described above

9 = Vigorous activity: run 20 to 25 miles per week or spend 7 to 8 hours per week in comparable physical activity as described above

10 = Vigorous activity: run more than 25 miles per week or spend more than 8 hours per week in comparable physical activity as described above

Modified from Jackson AS, Blair SN, Mahar MT, Wier LT, Ross RM, Stuteville JE. Prediction of functional aerobic capacity without exercise testing. *Med Sci Sports Exerc.* 1990;22(6):863-870.

POSITIVE FINDINGS

- Below average predicted VO_2max values

SPECIAL CONSIDERATION

- This equation is most applicable to healthy, active males and females

REFERENCES

1. Bradshaw DI, George JD, Hyde A, et al. An accurate VO_2max nonexercise regression model for 18-65 year-old adults. *Res Q Exerc Sport.* 2005;76:426-432.

DUKE ACTIVITY STATUS INDEX

ACTION

- To predict VO_2peak in clients with heart disease, complete the Duke Activity Status Index (DASI)

Table 5-13

THE DUKE ACTIVITY STATUS INDEX

Check each of the following tasks you can do.

✓	*Can you:*	*Weight*
	Take care of yourself (dress, bathe, or use the toilet?)	2.75
	Walk indoors, such as around your house?	1.75
	Walk a block or two on level ground?	2.75
	Climb a flight of stairs or walk uphill?	5.00
	Run a short distance?	8.00
	Do light work around the house like dusting or washing dishes?	2.70
	Do moderate work around the house like vacuuming, sweeping floors, or moving heavy furniture?	3.50
	Do heavy work around the house like scrubbing floors, or lifting or moving heavy furniture?	8.00
	Do yard work like raking leaves, weeding, or pushing a power mower?	4.50
	Have sexual relations?	5.25
	Participate in moderate recreational activities like golf, bowling, dancing, doubles tennis, or throwing a baseball or football?	6.00
	Participate in strenuous sports like swimming, singles tennis, football, basketball, or skiing?	7.50
	VO_2peak (mL/kg/min) = [0.43 × (sum of weights)] + 9.6	Σ

Used with permission from Hlatky MA, Boineau RE, Higginbotham MB, et al. A brief self-administered questionnaire to determine functional capacity (the Duke Activity Status Index). *Am J Cardiol.* 1989;64(10):651-654.

- Clinician adds weights, uses equation, and calculates VO_2peak

NORMAL FINDINGS
- The higher the calculated peak VO_2 value, the better the client's functional capability

POSITIVE FINDINGS
- VO_2peak <17.5 mL/kg/min suggests functional independence limitations

SPECIAL CONSIDERATIONS
- Better assessment for those >5 MET max[1]
- The DASI is reliable, valid, and responsive to clinical changes[2]
- The DASI predicts VO_2peak in those with coronary artery disease, congestive heart failure, and chronic pulmonary disease

REFERENCES
1. Hlatky MA, Boineau RE, Higginbotham MB, et al. A brief self-administered questionnaire to determine functional capacity (the Duke Activity Status Index). *Am J Cardiol.* 1989;64:651-654.
2. Alonso J, Permanyer-Miralda G, Cascant P, et al. Measuring functional status of chronic coronary clients: reliability, validity and responsiveness to clinical change of the reduced version of the Duke Activity Status Index (DASI). *Eur Heart J.* 1997;18:414-419.

SUBMAXIMAL EXERCISE

TWO-MINUTE WALK TEST

ACTION

- Cones placed in line 100 feet apart (or as far apart as possible within setting)
- Seated 10-minute rest; vital signs assessed
- Client instructed to walk as fast and as far as possible
- Use standard instructions and praise
  - ✧ Example: "You have completed 1 minute. You are doing well."
- Timing of test continues even if client stops
  - ✧ Place chairs at each end and in the middle of course
  - ✧ Discourage client from sitting down; may stop and stand to rest if needed
- Heart rate and rhythm recorded during test if not disruptive
- Record total distance walked in allotted time
- Measure pre- and post-test blood pressures
- Recorded speed can be converted into VO_2 cost

Table 5-14

CHARACTERISTICS OF THE 2-MINUTE WALK TEST

Safely Completed	Reproducible	Valid	Responsive to Change	Learning Effect
Frail elderly[1]	5-year-olds with cystic fibrosis[2]	Elderly rehabilitation[3]	Elderly rehabilitation[3]	
		Following cardiac surgery[4]	Following cardiac surgery[4]	
		Postpolio[5]		
				Transtibial amputation[6]
		Cardiac surgery[7]		
	Neurological impairment[8]	Neurological impairment[8]		

SPECIAL CONSIDERATIONS

- Actual VO_2 for specific walking speed can be predicted with the following equation[9]
    - VO_2 (mL·kg^{-1}·min^{-1}) = 0.1 (speed) + 3.5 mL·kg^{-1}·min^{-1}
- Equation valid for speeds between 1.9 and 3.7 mph
- 1 mph = 26.8 m/min^{-1}

REFERENCES

1. Brooks D, Davis AM, Naglie G. The feasibility of six-minute and two-minute walk tests in in-patient geriatric rehabilitation. *Can J Aging.* 2007;26:159-162.

2. Upton CJ, Tyrrell JC, Hiller EJ. Two-minute walking distance in cystic fibrosis. *Arch Dis Child.* 1988;63:1444-1448.

3. Brooks D, Davis AM, Naglie G. Validity of 3 physical performance measures in inpatient geriatric rehabilitation. *Arch Phys Med Rehabil.* 2006;1:105-110.

4. Brooks D, Parsons J, Tran D, et al. The two-minute walk test as a measure of functional capacity in cardiac surgery patients. *Arch Phys Med Rehabil.* 2004;85:1525-1530.

5. Stolwijk-Swüste JM, Beelen A, Lankhorst GJ, Nollet F; CARPA study group. SF-36 physical functioning scale and 2-minute walk test advocated as core qualifiers to evaluate physical functioning in patients with late-onset sequelae of poliomyelitis. *J Rehabil Med.* 2008;40;387-394.

6. Brooks D, Hunter JP, Parsons J, et al. Reliability of the two-minute walk test in individuals with transtibial amputation. *Arch Phys Med Rehabil.* 2002;83:1562-1565.

7. Brooks D, Parsons J, Tran D, et al. The two-minute walk test as a measure of functional capacity in cardiac surgery patients. *Arch Phys Med Rehabil.* 2004;9:1525-1530.

8. Rossier P, Wade DT. Validity and reliability comparison of 4 mobility measures in patients presenting with neurology impairment. *Arch Phys Med Rehabil.* 2001;82:9-13.

9. American College of Sports Medicine. *ACSM Guidelines for Exercise Testing and Prescription.* 7th ed. Philadelphia, PA: Lippincott Williams & Wilkins; 2006.

SIX-MINUTE WALK TEST

ACTION

- Explain that client should walk as far as possible in 6 minutes
- Client may slow down, stop, rest, restart as needed during the test
- Demonstrate how to walk the course, including turns
- Obtain baseline heart rate, blood pressure, oxygen saturation, and perceptual responses (perceived exertion, angina, claudication, dyspnea)
- Record laps, mark stopping point, measure distance walked during the test, and carefully observe active recovery
- Use available equations to predict expected 6-minute walk distances (6-MWD) in healthy adults (see page 231)

NORMAL FINDINGS

- >300 m elapsed distance in elderly or debilitated clients[1,2] (see Appendix A on page 264)
- 12- to 16-year-old Chinese adolescents walked 659.8 ± 58.1 m[3]
- Average or better than average predicted VO_2max (see Appendix A on page 264)

POSITIVE FINDINGS

- <300 m suggests increased risk of mortality in adult clients[1] (see Appendix A on page 264)
- <602 m suggests improvement needed for adolescents[2,3]
- Below average predicted VO_2max (see Appendix A on page 264)

SPECIAL CONSIDERATIONS

- Absolute contraindications[1]
    - ✧ Unstable angina or myocardial infarction within the last month
- Relative contraindications[1]
    - ✧ Resting HR >120 b/min
    - ✧ Resting SBP >180 mm Hg; resting DBP >100 mm Hg
- Standard encouragement should always be used[1]
    - ✧ "Looking good. You have 5 minutes to go."
    - ✧ "Keep it up. You have 4 minutes to go."

- ❖ "Looking good. You have 3 minutes to go."
- ❖ "Keep it up. You have 2 minutes to go."
- ❖ "Looking good. You have 1 minute to go."
- Widely used exercise evaluation tool with low morbidity/mortality[1,4]
- 6-MWT valid and reliable in adolescents (mean age = 14.2 ± 1.2 yrs)[3]
- 6-MWT correlates very highly (r = 0.96) with 12-minute test[5]
- 6-MWT generally elicits intensities within individual's training range
- ~≥7% learning effect, administer test at least twice (30-minute rest between tests), using best score for comparison[1]
- No discernible difference in indoor vs outdoor test
- Greater distance achieved on circular/oval vs straight, out and back courses
- Lower limit of normal for 6-MWD = 423 m and 355 m for healthy males and females (40 to 80 years old), respectively[6]

PREDICTED 6-MWD FOR 45 TO 85 YEARS OF AGE[7]

- Measure height, age, and BMI
    - ❖ Males: 6-MWD (meters) = 867 − [5.71 x age (yr)] + [1.03 x height (cm)]
    - ❖ Females: 6-MWD (meters) = 525 − [2.86 x age (yr)] +[2.71 x height (cm)] − (6.22 x BMI)
    - ❖ r^2= 0.40 and 0.43 for males and females, respectively

PREDICT PEAK VO$_2$ IN HEALTHY SUBJECTS, 50 TO 70 YEARS OLD[8]

- Measure distance and percentage of fat
- Peak VO_2 = 20.05 + 0.019 (maximal distance) − 0.278 (% fat)
- r = 0.81, r^2 = 0.66

PREDICT PEAK VO$_2$ IN CLIENTS WITH CONGESTIVE HEART FAILURE[9]

- Measure distance, weight, height, rate pressure product, and age
- Peak VO_2 = VO_2mL·kg^{-1}·min^{-1} = [0.02 x distance (m)] − [0.191 x age (yr)] − [0.07 x weight (kg)] + [0.09 x height (cm)] + [0.26 x RPP (x 10-3)] + 2.45
- r = 0.81, r^2 = 0.65 → r = 0.85, r^2 = 0.72

SUBMAXIMAL EXERCISE

Predict VO$_2$peak in Clients With End-Stage Lung Disease[10]

- Measure distance, age, and weight
- Peak VO$_2$ = 0.005 x distance (ft) – 0.162 x age (yr) + 0.05 x weight (kg) – 2.04 x forced vital capacity (L) + 2.45 x forced expiratory volume in 1 second (L) + 0.084 x diffusion capacity of carbon monoxide (mL·min·mm Hg) + 9.75
- $r = 0.76$, $r^2 = 0.58$ → $r = 0.83$, $r^2 = 0.89$

References

1. ATS Committee on Proficiency Standards for Clinical Pulmonary Function Laboratories. ATS statement: guidelines for the six-minute walk test. *Am J Respir Crit Care Med.* 2002;166:111-117.

2. Rostagno C, Olivo G, Comeglio M, et al. Prognostic value of 6-minute walk corridor test in patients with mild to moderate heart failure: comparison with other methods of functional evaluation. *Eur J Heart Fail.* 2003;5:247-252.

3. Li AM, Yin J, Yu CCW, et al. The six-minute walk test in healthy children: reliability and validity. *Eur Respir J.* 2005;25:1057-1060.

4. Solway S, Brooks D, Lacasse Y, et al. A qualitative systematic overview of the measurement properties of functional walk tests used in the cardiorespiratory domain. *Chest.* 2005;119:256-270.

5. Butland RJA, Pang J, Gross ER, et al. Two-, six-, and twelve-minute walking tests in respiratory disease. *Brit Med J.* 1982;824:1607-1608.

6. Enright PL, Sherrill DL. Reference equations for the six-minute walk in healthy adults. *Am J Crit Care Med.* 1998;158:1384-1387.

7. Jenkins S, Cecins N, Camarri B, Williams C, Thompson P, Eastwood P. Regression equations to predict 6-minute walk distance in middle-aged and elderly adults. *Physiotherapy Theory Pract.* 2009;25:516-522.

8. Swisher AK, Goldfarb AH. Use of the six-minute walk/run test to predict peak oxygen consumption in older adults. *Cardiopulm Phys Ther.* 1998;9:3-5.

9. Cahalin LP, Mathier MA, Semigran MJ, Dec GW, DiSalvo TG. The six-minute walk test predicts peak oxygen uptake and survival in patients with advanced heart failure. *Chest.* 1996;110:325-332.

10. Cahalin L, Pappagianopoulos P, Prevost S, Wain J, Ginns L. The relationship of the 6-min walk test to maximal oxygen consumption in transplant candidates with end-stage lung disease. *Chest.* 1995;108:452-459.

SUBMAXIMAL
EXERCISE

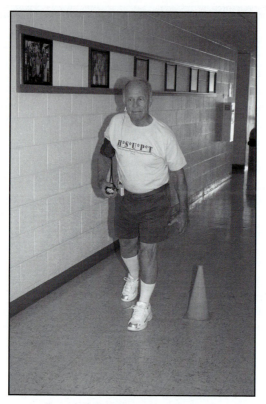

FIGURE 5-4. SIX-MINUTE WALK TEST.

SIX-MINUTE WALK TEST ON TREADMILL FOR YOUNGER ADULTS[1]

ACTION

- Measure body weight (kg) prior to the test
- Instruct client to walk as fast as possible on a treadmill set at 1% grade
- Client may adjust speed at any time
- Record total distance walked during the 6-minute test
- Obtain heart rate during last 15 seconds of the test
- Predict VO_2max (L·min^{-1})
    - ❖ VO_2max (L·min^{-1}) = {−1.732 + [weight (kg) x 0.049]} + {[distance (m) x 0.005]} + {[HR (beats/min) x 0.015]}, r= 0.87, (SEE 0.399)[1]
    - ❖ Multiply VO_2max by 1000, divide by body mass (kg) to predict VO_2max (mL·kg^{-1}·min^{-1})

NORMAL FINDINGS

- Mean = 47.01 mL·kg^{-1}·min^{-1} ± 6.68 (within 1 standard deviation)
- Use other normative data as needed (see Appendix A on page 264)
- Normal hemodynamic responses

POSITIVE FINDINGS

- Predicted VO_2max <40.33 mL·kg^{-1}·min^{-1} suggests aerobic training is needed
- Abnormal hemodynamic responses

SPECIAL CONSIDERATION

- Predictive equation for healthy young adults (29.5 mL·kg^{-1}·min^{-1} ± 9.9 years of age)

REFERENCE

1. Laskin JJ, Bundy S, Marron H, et al. Using a treadmill for the 6-minute walk test: reliability and validity. *J Cardiopulm Rehabil Prev.* 2007;27:407-410.

SUBMAXIMAL EXERCISE

TIMED ONE-MILE WALK

ACTION

- Walk 1 mile as quickly as possible; remain standing when finished
- Obtain immediate 15-second postexercise heart rate; calculate minute value
- Enter data in equation below and predict VO_2max
- $VO_2max = 132.853 - 0.1692$ (body mass in kg) $- 0.3877$ (age in years) $+ 6.315$ (gender: 0 = female, 1 = male) $- 3.2649$ (time in minutes) $- 0.1565$ (HR-final minute)[1]
- $r = 0.93$, SEE $= 5.0$ mL·kg^{-1}·min^{-1}
- Compare predicted VO_2max to normative data (see Table 5-3 on page 206)

NORMAL FINDINGS

- Average or above aerobic fitness
- Normal hemodynamic responses

POSITIVE FINDINGS

- Below average aerobic fitness
- Abnormal hemodynamic responses

SPECIAL CONSIDERATIONS

- Test most appropriate for 30 to 69 year olds,[1] not college students[2]
- As mentioned for previous tests, clients must avoid nicotine, caffeine, and other heart rate altering medications or products
- Clients must be appropriately screened and warned against running
- Clients should stretch following activity, then cool down
- Verbal encouragement should be standardized

REFERENCES

1. Kline GM, Porcari JP, Hintermeister R, et al. Estimation of VO_2max from a one-mile track walk, gender, age, and body weight. *Med Sci Sports Exerc.* 1987;19:253-259.
2. Dolgener FA, Hensley LD, Marsh JJ, Fjelstul JK. Validation of the Rockport Fitness Walking Test in college males and females. *Res Q Exerc Sport.* 1994;65:152-158.

SUBMAXIMAL EXERCISE

SEATED STEP TEST (SST)[1]

ACTION

- Sit in comfortable straight back chair
- Position step so that client's instep rests on top edge of step
- 6-, 12-, and 18-inch step benches are used

Table 5-15

SEATED STEP TEST WORKLOADS, STEP HEIGHTS, AND INTENSITY

Workload	Step Height (in)	METs
1	6	2.3
2	12	2.9
3	18	3.5
4	18	3.9

Adapted from Smith EL, Gilligan C. Physical activity for the older adult. *Phys Sportsmed.* 1983;11:91-101.

- Set metronome to 60 clicks/min or 15 steps per minute
- Client steps up and down with right leg, then left leg for 2 minutes
- Assess heart rate; if below 75% of maximum, test continues[1]
- Client steps for an additional 5 minutes at same workload
- Heart rate may be recorded each minute and blood pressure may be recorded every 2 minutes
- Procedure is repeated for 12-inch and 18-inch steps if heart rate remains below 75% predicted maximum
- The fourth workload requires client to flex his/her ipsilateral arm to horizontal as he/she steps

NORMAL FINDINGS

- In those not affected by cardiac medications, heart rate, SBP, rate of perceived exertion, or breathing frequency should be maintained or increased slightly with increasing workloads

SUBMAXIMAL EXERCISE

ABNORMAL FINDINGS

- A lack of increase or a decrease in physiological responses with increasing workloads in the unmedicated

SPECIAL CONSIDERATIONS

- Calibrate metronome and check step height prior to testing
- Heart rate and SBP responses may be blunted in those taking Beta antagonists
- Submaximal exercise and heart rate responses are reliable[2]
- Very safe test when properly administered in an elderly population[3]
- SST compares favorably with self-reported measures of functional status[3]
- Low-intensity test with workloads equivalent to household tasks
- Homebound women with moderate disabilities performed the SST[3]
- Nonambulatory can perform the SST[3]
- SST workloads may also serve as a "known intensity" workout

REFERENCES

1. Smith EL, Gilligan C. Physical activity for the older adult. *Phys Sportsmed.* 1983;11:91-101.
2. Tonino RP, Driscoll PA. Reliability of maximal and submaximal parameters of treadmill testing for the measurement of physical training in older persons. *J Gerontol.* 1988;43:101-104.
3. Simonsick E, Fried LP. Exercise tolerance and body composition. In: Guralnik JM, Fried LP, Simonsick EM, Kasper KD, Lafferty ME, eds. *The Women's Health and Aging Study: Health and Social Characteristics of Older Women With Disability.* Bethesda, MD: National Institute on Aging; 1995:106-117. NIH Publication No. 95-4009.

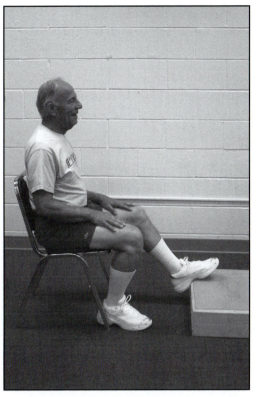

FIGURE 5-5. SEATED STEP TEST, 6 INCH.

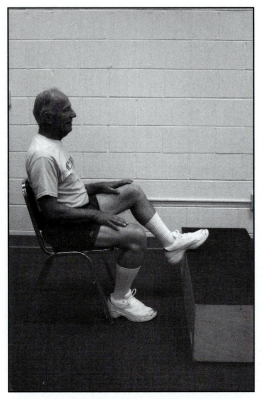

FIGURE 5-6. SEATED STEP TEST, 12 INCH.

SUBMAXIMAL
EXERCISE

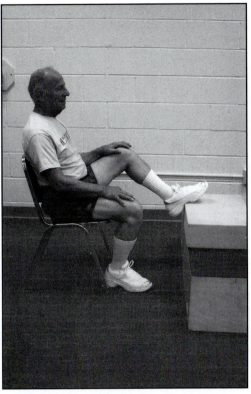

FIGURE 5-7. SEATED STEP TEST, 18 INCH.

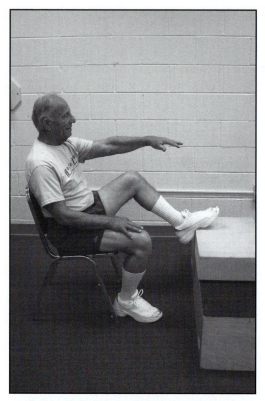

FIGURE 5-8. SEATED STEP TEST WITH ARMS,
18 INCH.

TECUMSEH STEP TEST

ACTION

- Use an 8-inch bench; explain and demonstrate test
- Metronome calibrated and set at 96 beats/minute (24 steps/minute)
  - ✧ Client steps "up-up, down-down, up-up, down-down" for 3 minutes
  - ✧ Either foot may be used to lead
- Assess standing heart rate immediately upon completion of the test, counting heartbeats from 30-60 seconds[1] of recovery
- Compare heart rate count to normative data[1,2]
- Normative sample of 5448 males and females, ages 10 to 69 years[1,2]

Table 5-16

TECUMSEH STEP TEST

Normative 30-60 second recovery heart beat counts after 1-min rest.

Classification	Out-standing	Good	Average	Fair	Poor
Men by Age					
20 - 29	34 - 40	41 - 44	45 - 47	48 - 51	52 - 59
30 - 39	35 - 41	42 - 45	46 - 47	48 - 51	52 - 59
40 - 49	37 - 42	43 - 46	47 - 49	50 - 53	54 - 60
50 - 59	37 - 43	44 - 47	48 - 49	50 - 53	54 - 62
60 - 69	35 - 41	42 - 46	47 - 49	50 - 52	53 - 59
Women by Age					
20 - 39	39 - 45	46 - 48	49 - 52	53 - 56	57 - 66
30 - 39	39 - 45	46 - 49	50 - 52	53 - 56	57 - 66
40 - 49	41 - 45	46 - 49	50 - 53	54 - 57	58 - 67
50 - 59	41 - 47	48 - 51	52 - 54	55 - 58	59 - 66
60 - 69	42 - 45	46 - 49	50 - 51	52 - 56	57 - 63

*Data based on heart rates measured 30-60 seconds after standard 3-min step test (using 8-inch step @ 24 steps/min.)

Adapted from Montoye HJ. *Physical Activity and Health: An Epidemiologic Study of an Entire Community.* Englewood Cliffs, NJ: Prentice-Hall; 1975.

NORMAL FINDINGS

- Average, good, and outstanding heart rate recovery responses

POSITIVE FINDINGS

- Fair and poor recovery heart rate response
- Heart rate or SBP failing to increase; other signs and symptoms as noted earlier

SPECIAL CONSIDERATIONS

- This test has an energy cost of 5.7 METs, which equals vigorous intensity for the average middle-aged American adult
- May be too difficult for sedentary adults

REFERENCES

1. Montoye HJ. *Physical Activity and Health: An Epidemiologic Study of an Entire Community.* Englewood Cliffs, NJ: Prentice-Hall; 1975.
2. Montoye HJ. Circulatory-respiratory fitness. In: Montoye HJ, ed. *Physical Fitness.* Indianapolis, IN: Phi Epsilon Kappa Fraternity; 1970. *An Introduction to Measurement in Physical Education;* vol 4.

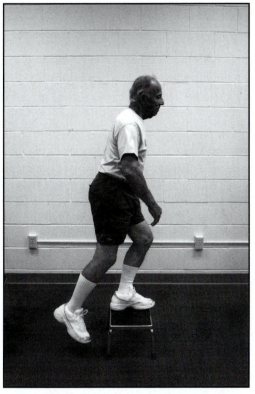

FIGURE 5-9. TECUMSEH STEP TEST.

YMCA STEP TEST[1,2]

ACTION

- Use a 12-inch bench; explain and demonstrate test
- Metronome calibrated and set at 96 beats/min (24 steps/min)
  - ✧ Client steps "up-up, down-down, up-up, down-down" for 3 min
  - ✧ Either foot may be used to lead
- Feet must be flat on the floor or the step during the test
- A full upright position must be maintained during the test
- Sit immediately upon test completion or cessation
- Within 10 sec of test termination, measure heart rate for 1 min
- Blood pressure may be measured after postexercise heart rate
- Heart rate response is compared against normative data

NORMAL FINDINGS

Table 5-17

YMCA STEP TEST RECOVERY HEART RATES AND FITNESS CATEGORY FOR MEN[2]

Age (yrs)	18-25	26-35	36-45	46-55	56-65	65+
Excellent	50-76	51-76	49-76	56-82	60-77	59-81
Good	79-84	79-85	80-88	87-93	86-94	87-92
Above Avg.	88-93	88-94	92-98	95-101	97-100	94-102
Average	95-100	96-102	100-105	103-111	103-109	104-110
Below Avg.	102-107	104-110	108-113	113-119	111-117	114-118
Poor	111-119	114-121	116-124	121-126	119-128	121-126
Very Poor	124-157	126-161	130-163	131-159	131-154	130-151

Adapted from Golding LA, ed. *YMCA Fitness Testing and Assessment Manual,* 4th ed. Champaign, IL: YMCA of the USA; 2000.

Table 5-18

YMCA STEP TEST RECOVERY HEART RATES AND FITNESS CATEGORY FOR WOMEN[2]

Age (yrs)	18-25	26-35	36-45	46-55	56-65	65+
Excellent	52-81	58-80	51-84	63-91	60-92	70-92
Good	85-93	85-92	89-96	95-101	97-103	96-101
Above Avg.	96-102	95-101	100-104	104-110	106-111	104-111
Average	104-110	104-110	107-112	113-118	113-118	116-121
Below Avg.	113-120	113-119	115-120	120-124	119-127	123-126
Poor	121-131	122-129	124-132	126-132	129-135	128-133

Adapted from Golding LA, ed. *YMCA Fitness Testing and Assessment Manual,* 4th ed. Champaign, IL: YMCA of the USA; 2000.

- Increased heart rate, SBP, rate of perceived exertion, respiratory frequency
- 1-minute heart rate responses that are average or above

ABNORMAL FINDINGS
- Signs and symptoms of exercise intolerance
  - ✧ Heart rate or SBP failing to increase
  - ✧ Diastolic blood pressure increasing or decreasing to >100 mm Hg

SPECIAL CONSIDERATIONS
- The intensity of this test is approximately 7.4 MET level, which is close to maximal for most healthy, middle-aged American adults
- Test retest reliability is high (r = 0.90)[2]

REFERENCES
1. Kasch FW, Phillips WH, Ross WD, Carter JE, Boyer JL. A comparison of maximal oxygen uptake by treadmill and step-test procedures. *J Appl Physiol.* 1966;21:1387-1398.
2. Golding LA, ed. *YMCA Fitness Testing and Assessment Manual,* 4th ed. Champaign, IL: YMCA of the USA; 2000.

SUBMAXIMAL EXERCISE

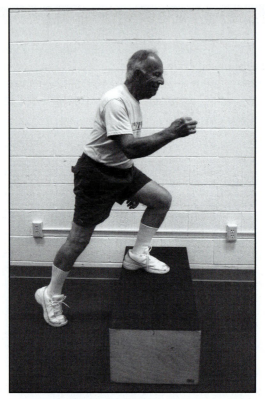

FIGURE 5-10. YMCA STEP TEST.

ASTRAND-RYHMING CYCLE ERGOMETER TEST

ACTION

- Use a calibrated cycle ergometer
- ~10° knee flexion angle with one foot fully extended on pedal
- Measure resting heart rate and blood pressure
- Calculate heart rates between 50% and 85% heart rate reserve
- Tape blood pressure cuff in place
- Select initial workload for subject[1]

Table 5-19

WORKLOAD SELECTION TABLE FOR ASTRAND CYCLE ERGOMETER TEST[2]

	Unconditioned	*Conditioned*
Males	300 or 600 kg·m·min^{-1}	600 or 900 kg·m·min^{-1}
Females	300 or 450 kg·m·min^{-1}	450 or 600 kg·m·min^{-1}

Adapted from American College of Sports Medicine. *ACSM Guidelines for Exercise Testing and Prescription.* 7th ed. Philadelphia, PA: Lippincott Williams & Wilkins; 2006.

- Calibrate metronome for 100 clicks per minute, pedal at 50 rpm
  - ✧ With each metronome beat, one foot should be in down position
- Visual feedback from speedometer may be used
- Proper pedaling rate must be constantly reinforced (see Figure 5-11 on page 246)
- Record heart rate each minute of the test, average minutes 5 and 6
  - ✧ Females and males must achieve heart rates of 122 and 120 beats/minute[1], respectively
- Obtain exercise and recovery blood pressure
- On nomogram: (see Figure 5-12 on page 247)
  - ✧ Mark mean heart rate (minutes 5 and 6) on left scale and final workload on right scale[1,2]
  - ✧ Draw a line between these 2 points and note where line crosses the predicted VO_2max line[1]

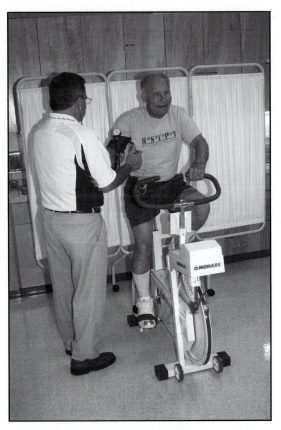

FIGURE 5-11. ASTRAND-RYHMING
CYCLE ERGOMETER TEST.

- Using the VO_2 (L·min^{-1}) value from the nomogram and age (yrs), compute VO_2max using gender specific regression equations below[3]
  - ♀ VO_2max (L·min^{-1}) = [0.348 (X1) − 0.035 (X2)] + 3.011
  - ♂ VO_2max (L·min^{-1}) = [0.302 (X1) − 0.019 (X2)] + 1.593
    - ⌐ X1 = VO_2 from nomogram; X2 = age (yrs)

NORMAL FINDINGS

- At or above average based on gender (see Appendix A on page 264)

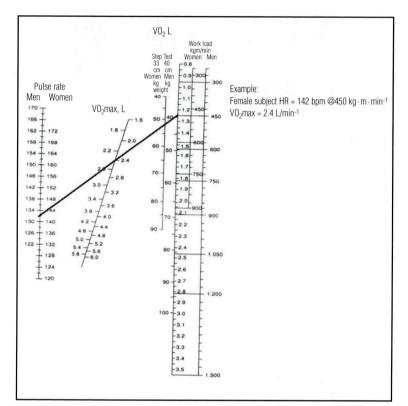

FIGURE 5-12. SAMPLE NOMOGRAM PLOT FOR ASTRAND-RYHMING CYCLE ERGOM-
ETER TEST. (USED WITH PERMISSION FROM ASTRAND PO, RYHMING I. A NOMO-
GRAM FOR CALCULATION OF AEROBIC CAPACITY [PHYSICAL FITNESS] FROM PULSE RATE
DURING SUBMAXIMAL WORK. *J APPL PHYSIOL.* 1954;7:218-221.)

ABNORMAL FINDINGS

- Below average based on gender (see Appendix A on page 264)

SPECIAL CONSIDERATIONS

- 50 rpm x 6 m/rev x 1 kg = 300 kg·m·min^{-1}
  300 kg·m·min^{-1} ÷ 6 = 50 watts
- Test is valid[3-5] and reliable[5]
- VO$_2$max predicted via cycle ergometry may underestimate treadmill VO$_2$max by up to 15% in walkers and runners
- Age-related correction factor of Astrand is not used with equations above

REFERENCES

1. Astrand PO, Ryhming I. A nomogram for calculation of aerobic capacity (physical fitness) from pulse rate during submaximal work. *J Appl Physiol.* 1954;7:218-221.

2. American College of Sports Medicine. *ACSM Guidelines for Exercise Testing and Prescription.* 7th ed. Philadelphia, PA: Lippincott Williams & Wilkins; 2006.

3. Siconolfi SF, Cullinane EM, Carleton RA, Thompson PD. Assessing VO_2max in epidemiologic studies: modification of the Astrand-Ryhming test. *Med Sci Sports Exerc.* 1982;14:335-338.

4. Cink RE, Thomas TR. Validity of the Astrand-Ryhming nomogram for predicting maximal oxygen intake. *Brit J Sports Med.* 1981;15:182-185.

5. Wilmore JH, Roby FB, Stanforth PR, et al. Ratings of perceived exertion, heart rate, and power output in predicting maximal oxygen uptake during submaximal cycle ergometry. *Phys Sports Med.* 1986;14:133-143.

SUBMAXIMAL EXERCISE

YMCA CYCLE ERGOMETER TEST

ACTION

- Use a calibrated cycle ergometer
- ~10° knee flexion angle with one foot fully extended on pedal
- Measure resting heart rate and blood pressure
- Calculate heart rates between 50% and 85% heart rate reserve
- Tape blood pressure cuff in place
- 1st stage: subject pedals against 0.5 kg resistance at 50 rpm (metronome = 100 beats/minute^{-1}) for 3 minutes
- Heart rate must steady-state (±5 beats/minute) for minutes 2 and 3 of each 3-minute stage
- If no steady-state, pedal extra minute, average minutes 3 and 4; repeat until steady-state is met
- 2nd, 3rd, and 4th stages are based on average heart rate response from previous stage

---

Table 5-20

YMCA CYCLE ERGOMETER TEST WORKLOADS

Stage 1	Heart Rate after Stage 1	Stage 2	Stage 3	Stage 4
0.5 kg →	<80 →	2.5 kg →	3.0 kg →	3.5 kg
0.5 kg →	80-89 →	2.0 kg →	2.5 kg →	3.0 kg
0.5 kg →	90-100 →	1.5 kg →	2.0 kg →	2.5 kg
0.5 kg →	>100 →	1.0 kg →	1.5 kg →	2.0 kg

To determine actual work load (kg·m·min^{-1}), multiply the resistance (kg) by the pedaling frequency (most commonly 50 rpm) by the distance the flywheel travels in 1 revolution (6 meters).

Modified from Golding LA, ed. *YMCA Fitness Testing and Assessment Manual,* 4th ed. Champaign, IL: YMCA of the USA; 2000.

- One stage must provide steady-state heart rate >110 beats/minute and a second stage must provide a steady-state heart rate <150 beats/minute

- To predict VO$_2$max using graphs (Figures 5-13 and 5-14)
    - ✧ Plot horizontal line identifying predicted max heart rate (220 – age)
    - ✧ Plot steady-state heart rate (at minute 2 and 3) for each stage
    - ✧ Draw a line through these average heart rates at each stage
    - ✧ Steady-state line will bisect the predicted maximum heart rate line
    - ✧ Draw a vertical line downward from this intersection
    - ✧ Predicted VO$_2$max can be found along the x-axis
    - ✧ VO$_2$max (L/min) x 1000 → mL/min ÷ body weight (kg) → mL·kg^{-1}·min^{-1}

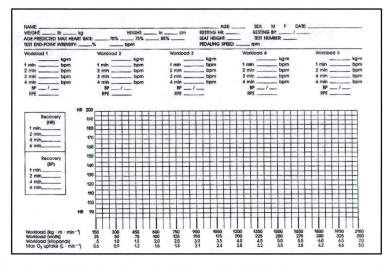

FIGURE 5-13. PREDICTION OF VO$_2$MAX/MAX METS FROM STEADY-STATE HEART RATE. (USED WITH PERMISSION FROM GOLDING LA, ED. *YMCA FITNESS TESTING AND ASSESSMENT MANUAL*, 4TH ED. CHAMPAIGN, IL: YMCA OF THE USA; 2000.)

SUBMAXIMAL EXERCISE

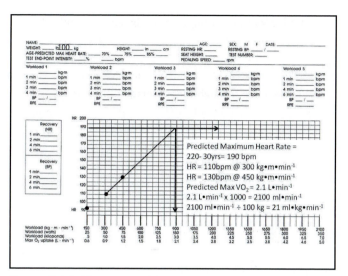

FIGURE 5-14. HEART RATE-MET VO$_2$ PREDICTION EXAMPLE. (USED WITH PERMISSION FROM GOLDING LA, ED. *YMCA FITNESS TESTING AND ASSESSMENT MANUAL,* 4TH ED. CHAMPAIGN, IL: YMCA OF THE USA; 2000.)

NORMAL FINDINGS

- VO$_2$max at or above average based on gender (see Appendix A on page 264)

ABNORMAL FINDINGS

- VO$_2$max below average based on gender (see Appendix A on page 264)

SINGLE-STAGE TREADMILL TEST

ACTION
- Obtain history and perform usual pre-exercise assessment
- Set treadmill grade at 0%, speed from 2.0 to 4.5 mph
- Calculate exercise heart rates equivalent to 50% and 70% of maximum
- Walking speed should elicit heart rates between 50% and 70% of maximum
- Walk for 4 minutes, measuring heart rate each minute
- Increase grade to 5% and walk for 4 minutes measuring heart rate
- Calculate VO_2max[1]
- VO_2max = [15.1 + 21.8 x speed (mph)] − [0.327 x heart rate (bpm)] − [0.263 x speed (mph) x age (yrs)] + [0.00504 x heart rate x age (yrs)] + [5.98 x gender (0 = female, 1 =male)]

NORMAL FINDINGS
- VO_2max at or above 50% based on gender (see Appendix A on page 264)
- Normal hemodynamic responses

ABNORMAL FINDINGS
- VO_2max below 50% based on gender (see Appendix A on page 264)
- Abnormal hemodynamic responses

SPECIAL CONSIDERATION
- Valid and reliable test (r = 0.86, SEE = 4.85 mL/kg/min^{-1})[1]

REFERENCE
1. Ebbeling CB, Ward A, Puleo EM, et al. Development of a single-stage submaximal treadmill walking test. *Med Sci Sports Exerc.* 1991;23:966-973.

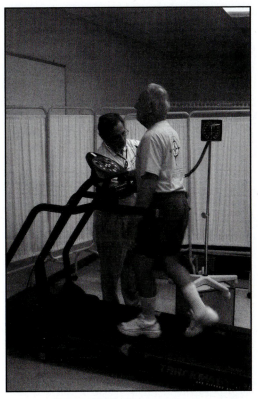

FIGURE 5-15. TREADMILL TEST.

NAUGHTON TREADMILL PROTOCOL

ACTION

- Obtain history and perform usual pre-exercise assessment
- Instruct client to walk or run during each 3-minute stage
- Record steady-state heart rate, blood pressure, and rate of perceived exertion

Table 5-21

NAUGHTON TREADMILL PROTOCOL[1]

Stage	% Grade	Speed (MPH)	VO$_2$max (mL•kg^{-1}•min^{-1})
1	0	2	7.0
2	3.5	2	10.5
3	7.0	2	14.0
4	10.5	2	17.5
5	14.0	2	21.0
6	17.5	2	24.5
7	12.5	3	28.0
8	15.0	3	31.5
9	17.5	3	35.0

Modified from Altug Z, Hoffman JL, Martin JL. *Manual of Clinical Exercise Testing, Prescription, and Rehabilitation.* Norwalk, CT: Appleton-Lange; 1993.

- Draw a horizontal line representing predicted max heart rate
- To predict VO$_2$max using graphs
  - ✧ Plot horizontal line identifying predicted max heart rate (220 – age)
  - ✧ Plot steady-state heart rate (at minute 2 and 3) for stages where heart rate was >110 and <150 beats/minute
  - ✧ Draw a line through average heart rates at each stage
  - ✧ Steady-state line bisects the predicted maximum heart rate line
  - ✧ Draw vertical line downward from this intersection
  - ✧ Predicted VO$_2$max in METs found along the x-axis

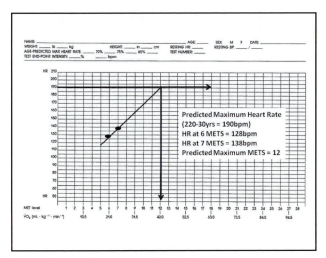

NAME: _____
WEIGHT: ____ lb ____ kg   HEIGHT: ____ in ____ cm   RESTING HR: ____
AGE-PREDICTED MAX HEART RATE: ____ 70% ____ 75% ____ 85% ____   TEST NUMBER: ____
TEST END-POINT INTENSITY: ____% ____ bpm

AGE: ____   SEX: M   F   DATE: _____
RESTING BP: ____ / ____

Predicted Maximum Heart Rate
(220-30yrs = 190bpm)
HR at 6 METS = 128bpm
HR at 7 METS = 138bpm
Predicted Maximum METS = 12

FIGURE 5-16. HEART RATE-MET VO$_2$ PREDICTION EXAMPLE. (USED WITH PERMISSION FROM ALTUG Z, HOFFMAN JL, MARTIN JL. *MANUAL OF CLINICAL EXERCISE TESTING, PRESCRIPTION, AND REHABILITATION.* NORWALK, CT: APPLETON-LANGE; 1993.)

NORMAL FINDINGS

- Appropriate hemodynamic responses and VO$_2$max average or better (see Table 5-3 on page 206)

POSITIVE FINDINGS

- Inappropriate hemodynamic responses and below average VO$_2$max (see Table 5-3 on page 206)-

SPECIAL CONSIDERATIONS

- Low initial intensity with 1-MET increases per 3-minute stage
- Optimal treadmill protocol for those who can walk because of low initial intensity and 1-MET increments
- Reliable in clients with heart transplants (r = 0.83)[2]
- Learning effect demonstrated at submaximal intensity of 80%; practice trials should be encouraged[3]
- Most widely used protocol in clients with heart failure[4]

REFERENCES

1. Altug Z, Hoffman JL, Martin JL. *Manual of Clinical Exercise Testing, Prescription, and Rehabilitation.* Norwalk, CT: Appleton-Lange; 1993.

2. Lewis ME, Newall C, Townend JN, Hill SL, Bonser RS. Incremental shuttle walk test in the assessment of patients for heart transplantation. *Heart.* 2001;86:183-187.

3. Russell SD, McNeer FR, Beere PA, Logan LJ, Higginbotham MB. Improvement in the mechanical efficiency of walking: an explanation for the "placebo effect" seen during repeated exercise testing of patients with heart failure. *Am Heart J.* 1998;135:107-114.

4. Kleber FX, Waurick P, Winterhalter M. CPET in heart failure. *Eur Heart J.* 2004;6:18-25.

WHEELCHAIR TEST

ACTION
- Obtain history and perform usual pre-exercise assessment (BP, HR, height, weight, and age)
- Outfit client with heart rate monitor
- Explain and demonstrate test
    - ✧ Wheel around a 400-meter outdoor[1] or 0.1-mile indoor track[2] as far as possible in 12 minutes
- Offer standard verbal encouragement

NORMAL FINDINGS
- HR, ventilation, BP increase during test
- Average or above average distance and predicted VO_2max scores

---

Table 5-22

WHEELCHAIR TEST NORMS

Indoor Test[2]		Outdoor Test[1]		
Distance (miles)	VO_2max mL·kg⁻¹·min⁻¹	Distance (miles)	VO_2max mL·kg⁻¹·min⁻¹	Fitness Level
<0.63	<7.7	<0.62	<12	Poor
0.6-0.86	7.7-14.5	.62-.87	13-17	Below average
0.87-1.35	14.6-29.1	.87-1.06	18-28	Average
1.36-1.59	29.2-36.2	1.06-1.24	28-35	Good
≥1.60	>36.3	>1.24	> 36	Excellent

Modified from Rhodes EC, McKenzie DC, Coutts KD, Rogers AR. A field test for the prediction of aerobic capacity in male paraplegics and quadriplegics. *Can J Appl Sport Sci.* 1981;6:182-186 and Franklin BA, Swantek KI, Grais SL, Johnstone KS, Gordon S, Timmis GC. Field test estimation of maximal oxygen consumption in wheelchair users. *Arch Phys Med Rehabil.* 1990;71:574-578.

POSITIVE FINDINGS
- Below average distance and predicted VO_2max scores

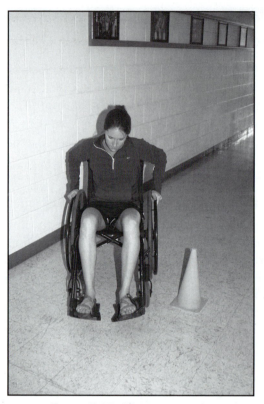

FIGURE 5-17. WHEELCHAIR TEST.

SUBMAXIMAL EXERCISE

SPECIAL CONSIDERATIONS

- All normative data were derived on male wheelchair users
- Arm-cycle VO_2max and wheelchair propulsion distances were highly correlated for the outdoor (r = 0.88) and indoor tests (r = 0.84)

REFERENCES

1. Rhodes EC, McKenzie DC, Coutts KD, Rogers AR. A field test for the prediction of aerobic capacity in male paraplegics and quadriplegics. *Can J Appl Sport Sci.* 1981;6:182-186.
2. Franklin BA, Swantek KI, Grais SL, Johnstone KS, Gordon S, Timmis GC. Field test estimation of maximal oxygen consumption in wheelchair users. *Arch Phys Med Rehabil.* 1990;71:574-578.

THE TALK TEST
(INDIRECT ASSESSMENT OF ANAEROBIC THRESHOLD)

ACTION
- Measure during progressive exercise test or at set intensity[1]
- Client reads the Pledge of Allegiance out loud[1]
- Ask client if they can speak comfortably[1-3]
  - ✧ Possible answers are "Yes," "I'm not sure," or "No"[1-3]

NORMAL FINDINGS
- Exercise intensity recommendations for general public at a comfortable speaking level
- Competitive athletes typically exercise below, at, and above a comfortable speaking level

ABNORMAL FINDINGS
- Unless there is a sport-specific purpose, most adults do not need to exercise at an intensity beyond a comfortable speaking level

Table 15-23

FINDINGS[1,2]

Possible Responses	Relation to Ventilatory Threshold	Group[3,4]
Yes	Below	College students, cardiac clients
I'm unsure	At or below	College students, cardiac clients
No	Above	College students, cardiac clients

Other exercise intensity data should also be gathered[2]

SPECIAL CONSIDERATIONS
- Identifying where speech becomes uncomfortable is a marker of the ventilatory threshold
- Ventilatory threshold often precedes myocardial ischemia in cardiac clients[4]

- It does not need to be exceeded in healthy persons during fitness training
- The Talk Test may be a highly consistent method of exercise prescription in college students on the cycle ergometer and treadmill[3]
- Affirmative and equivocal answers fall within normal heart rate and relative VO_2max exercise prescription intensities[4]

REFERENCES

1. Dehart-Beverley M, Foster C, Porcari JP, Fater DCW, Mikat RP. Relationship between the talk test and ventilatory threshold. *Clin Exerc Physiol.* 2000;2:34-38.

2. Voelker SA, Foster C, Porcari JP, Skemp KM, Brice G, Backes R. Relationship between the talk test and ventilatory threshold in cardiac patients. *Clin Exerc Physiol.* 2002;4:120-123.

3. Persinger R, Foster C, Gibson M, Fater DC, Porcari JP. Consistency of the talk test for exercise prescription. *Med Sci Sports Exerc.* 2004;36:1632-1636.

4. Meyer K, Samek L, Pinchas A, Baier M, Betz P, Roskamm H. Relationship between ventilatory threshold and onset of ischaemia in ECG during stress testing. *Eur Heart J.* 1995;16:623-630.

SUBMAXIMAL
EXERCISE

CALCULATING TARGET HEART RATES

PREDICT MAXIMAL HEART RATE (PMHR)

- 220 – age = predicted maximum heart rate

CALCULATE TARGET HEART RATES

- Method 1: Using resting heart rate
  - ✧ Calculate PMHR
  - ✧ Measure resting heart rate (RHR)
  - ✧ Select exercise intensity
    - ⅄ 40% for very ill or debilitated clients
    - ⅄ 50% for less debilitated clients
    - ⅄ >50% for most sedentary individuals
    - ⅄ <85% for all individuals
  - ✧ Target HR = [(PMHR – RHR) x intensity] + resting HR
  - ✧ Special considerations
    - ⅄ This method is usually less conservative than Method 2
    - ⅄ Intensity with this method is equivalent to the same percentage of maximum oxygen consumption.
- Method 2: Straight percentage method
  - ✧ PMHR x intensity
- Method 3: Heart rate plus method
  - ✧ RHR + 20 beats/minute[1]
    - ⅄ For clients with recent myocardial infarction or any client for whom there is extreme concern or risk
  - ✧ RHR + 30 beats/minute[1]
    - ⅄ For clients that have been revascularized (coronary artery bypass graft; stent)

EXAMPLE

- Client 1: Apparently healthy individual
- 50 years of age, RHR = 70 beats/minute
- PMHR = 170 beats/minute (220 – 50)

Method 1

- [(PMHR – RHR) x intensity] + resting HR
- [(170 – 70) x .7] + 70

SUBMAXIMAL
EXERCISE

- $[(100) \times .7] + 70$
- Target HR = 140 beats/minute

Method 2

- PMHR x intensity
- 170 x 0.70
- Target HR = 119 beats/minute

Early Rehabilitation (Hospitalized Client)

- RHR + 20 beats/minute[1]
- Target HR = 70 + 20 = 90 beats/minute

Less Severe Heart Condition

- Client 1 has chest pain, visits the ER, and receives a stent
- RHR + 30 beats/minute[1]
- Target HR = 70 + 30 = 100 beats/minute

REFERENCE

1. American College of Sports Medicine. *ACSM Guidelines for Exercise Testing and Prescription.* 7th ed. Philadelphia, PA: Lippincott Williams & Wilkins; 2006.

SUBMAXIMAL
EXERCISE

Appendices

APPENDIX A
MAXIMAL AEROBIC POWER

PERCENTILE VALUES FOR MAXIMAL AEROBIC POWER IN MEN (mL·kg^{-1}min^{-1})

Percentile	Age				
	20-29	30-39	40-49	50-59	60+
90	51.4	50.4	48.2	45.3	42.5
80	48.2	46.2	44.1	41.0	38.1
70	46.8	44.6	41.8	38.5	35.3
60	44.2	42.4	39.9	36.7	33.6
50	42.5	41.0	38.1	35.2	31.8
40	41.0	38.9	36.7	33.8	30.2
30	39.5	37.4	35.1	32.3	28.7
20	37.1	35.4	33.0	30.2	26.5
10	34.5	32.5	30.9	28.0	23.1

PERCENTILE VALUES FOR MAXIMAL AEROBIC POWER IN WOMEN (mL·kg^{-1}min^{-1})

Percentile	Age				
	20-29	30-39	40-49	50-59	60+
90	44.2	41.0	39.5	35.2	35.2
80	41.0	38.6	36.3	32.3	31.2
70	38.1	36.7	33.8	30.9	29.4
60	36.7	34.6	32.3	29.4	27.2
50	35.2	33.8	30.9	28.2	25.8
40	33.8	32.3	29.5	26.9	24.5
30	32.3	30.5	28.3	25.5	23.8
20	30.6	28.7	26.5	24.3	22.8
10	28.4	26.5	25.1	22.3	20.8

Adapted from: *ACSM's Guidelines for Exercise Testing and Exercise Prescription.* 7th ed. Philadelphia, PA: Lippincott, Williams, & Wilkins; 2006.

APPENDIX B
MONARK CYCLE ERGOMETER CALIBRATION[1]

ACTION

- Mechanical cycle ergometers must be calibrated and clients must keep proper cadence
- To calibrate leg cycle ergometers:
  - ✧ Disconnect resistance belt
  - ✧ "0" on panel must line up with pendulum
  - ✧ If not, adjust panel via wing nut until aligned
  - ✧ Hang 4 kg weight from hook and make sure the pendulum lines up with numbers on panel
  - ✧ If not, turn adjustment screw with screwdriver
  - ✧ Recheck "0"

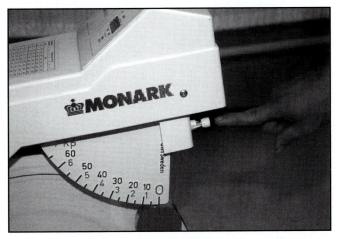

FIGURE B-1. CYCLE CALIBRATION (POINTING AT WING NUT).

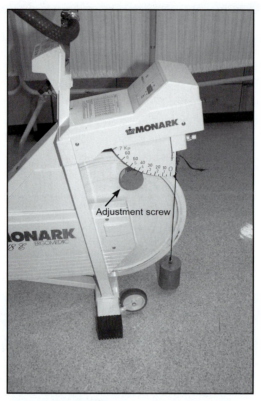

FIGURE B-2. CYCLE CALIBRATION
(HANG CALIBRATION WEIGHT).

REFERENCE

1. Astrand PO. *Work Tests With the Bicycle Ergometer*. Varberg, Sweden: Monark Crescent AB; 1988:14.

APPENDIX C
TREADMILL CALIBRATION

ACTION

- Speed calibration
    - ✧ Measure entire belt length
    - ✧ Mark belt "start point" with tape
    - ✧ Manually push belt around (Figure C-1) so that entire belt length is measured
    - ✧ Measure right side, left side, and middle belt length twice and average
    - ✧ Mark treadmill start point on side of treadmill
    - ✧ Start treadmill at specific speed
    - ✧ Start stopwatch when belt start point passes treadmill start point
    - ✧ Stop stopwatch when belt passes specific point on treadmill for the 10th complete revolution
    - ✧ Rev/min = 600/10 rev time(s)
    - ✧ MPH = belt length (in) x #rev/min ÷ 1056
        - ⅄ 1056 = conversion of inches per minute to miles per hour
- Adjustments
    - ✧ If calculated speed is >±0.5 mph different than speed on faceplate, make appropriate adjustments
        - ⅄ Usually via a calibration adjustment screw within a small opening in the front of the control panel or call service technician
    - ✧ Repeat calibration procedure at several different speeds to ascertain accuracy across commonly used protocols in your facility
    - ✧ Keep records of calibration checks
- Elevation or grade calibration (Figures C-2 and C-3)
    - ✧ If floor and treadmill are level (protractor angle = 0°)
        - ⅄ Test several commonly used grades throughout the range
    - ✧ Testing grade calibration (simple method)
        - ⅄ Use protractor commonly available in local stores

⅄   45°/100% = X°/selected % grade

⅄   Use 10% grade, which will yield 4.5°

⅄   If actual elevation is >0.5% different than faceplate value, make appropriate adjustments or contact service technicians

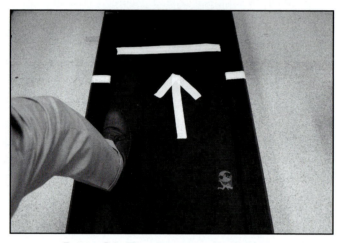

FIGURE C-1. TREADMILL SPEED CALIBRATION.

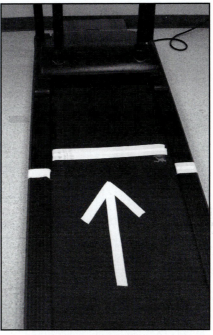

FIGURE C-2. TREADMILL LEVEL.

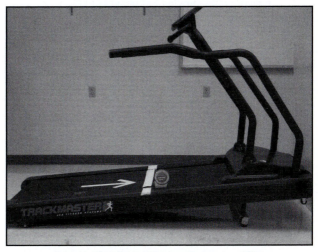

FIGURE C-3. TREADMILL ELEVATION = 10%,
PROTRACTOR ANGLE = 4.5°.

APPENDIX D
PREDICTION OF VO₂MAX/MAX METS FROM STEADY-STATE HEART RATE

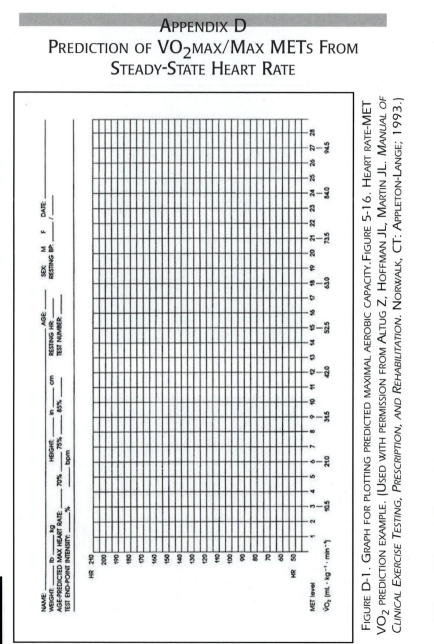

FIGURE D-1. GRAPH FOR PLOTTING PREDICTED MAXIMAL AEROBIC CAPACITY. FIGURE 5-16. HEART RATE-MET VO₂ PREDICTION EXAMPLE. (USED WITH PERMISSION FROM ALTUG Z, HOFFMAN JL, MARTIN JL. *MANUAL OF CLINICAL EXERCISE TESTING, PRESCRIPTION, AND REHABILITATION*. NORWALK, CT: APPLETON-LANGE; 1993.)

APPENDIX E
YMCA HR-VO₂MAX CHART

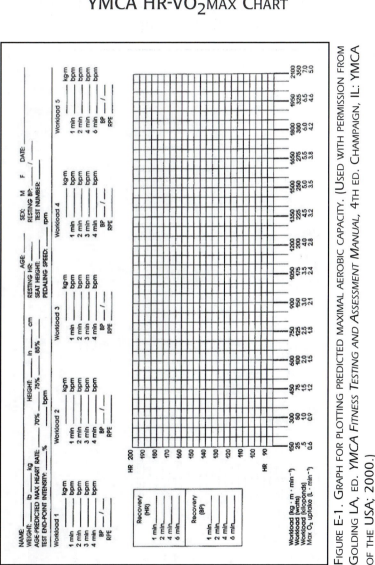

FIGURE E-1. GRAPH FOR PLOTTING PREDICTED MAXIMAL AEROBIC CAPACITY. (USED WITH PERMISSION FROM GOLDING LA, ED. *YMCA FITNESS TESTING AND ASSESSMENT MANUAL*, 4TH ED. CHAMPAIGN, IL: YMCA OF THE USA; 2000.)

APPENDIX F
ASTRAND-RYHMING NOMOGRAM

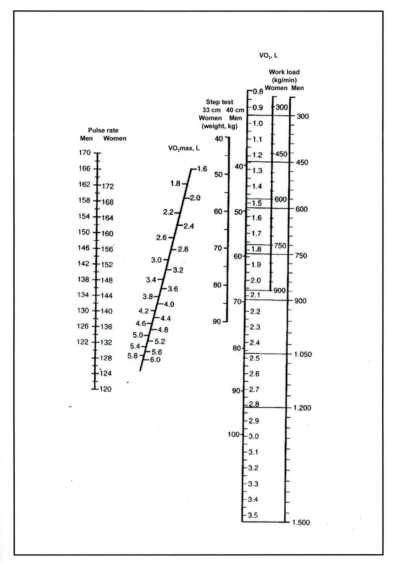

FIGURE F-1. (USED WITH PERMISSION FROM ASTRAND PO, RYHMING I. A NO-MOGRAM FOR CALCULATION OF AEROBIC CAPACITY [PHYSICAL FITNESS] FROM PULSE RATE DURING SUBMAXIMAL WORK. *J APPL PHYSIOL*. 1954;7:218-221.)

Index

Wait...There's More!

SLACK Incorporated's Health Care Books and Journals offers a wide selection of books in the field of Physical Therapy. We are dedicated to providing important works that educate, inform, and improve the knowledge of our customers. Don't miss out on our other informative titles that will enhance your collection.

Special Tests for Orthopedic Examination, Third Edition

Jeff G. Konin, PhD, ATC, PT; Denise L. Wiksten, PhD, ATC; Jerome A. Isear, Jr., MS, PT, ATC-L; Holly Brader, MPH, RN, BSN, ATC

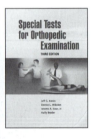

400 pp, Soft Cover, 2006, ISBN 13 978-1-55642-741-1, Order# 47417, **$43.95**

This clear and concise text has been used by thousands of students, clinicians, and rehab professionals and is available in its third edition. Concise and pocket-sized, this resource is an invaluable guide filled with the most current and practical clinical exam techniques used during an orthopedic examination, explaining more than 150 commonly used orthopedic special tests, including 11 new and modern tests.

Special Tests for Neurologic Examination

James R. Scifers, DScPT, PT, SCS, LAT, ATC

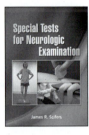

432 pp, Soft Cover, 2008, ISBN 13 978-1-55642-797-8, Order# 47972, **$43.95**

Ideal for students and clinicians to access quick clinical information, this comprehensive text offers invaluable evaluation and assessment tips and techniques for neurologic conditions commonly found in patients. Organized in an easy-to-use format, this text is the perfect guide for practicing clinical skills and reviewing for licensure and certification examinations.

Special Tests of the Cardiopulmonary, Vascular and Gastrointestinal Systems

Dennis G. O'Connell, PT, PhD, FACSM; Janelle K. O'Connell, PT, PhD, ATC-L; Martha R. Hinman, PT, EdD

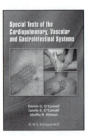

304 pp., Spiral Cover, 2011, ISBN 13 978-1-55642-966-8, Order# 49668, **$39.95**

Organized in a user-friendly format, this text provides a unique, compact, and concise summary of more than 95 special tests and exam procedures. In addition to the special tests categories, a submaximal exercise evaluation section has been added for clinicians who believe exercise is an excellent preventive and rehabilitative tool but who may be unfamiliar with the topic.

Please visit **www.slackbooks.com** to order any of the above titles!

24 Hours a Day...7 Days a Week!

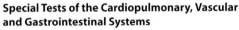

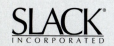